上海外国语大学教材基金资助

健康管理研究

李凌姝　张　丽　徐　林　金光辉　著

吉林出版集团股份有限公司｜全国百佳图书出版单位

版权所有　侵权必究

图书在版编目（CIP）数据

健康管理研究：汉英对照 / 李凌姝等著. -- 长春：吉林出版集团股份有限公司, 2022.2（2023.6重印）

ISBN 978-7-5731-1126-5

Ⅰ.①健… Ⅱ.①李… Ⅲ.①健康—卫生管理学—研究—汉、英 Ⅳ.① R19

中国版本图书馆 CIP 数据核字（2022）第 000131 号

JIANKANG GUANLI YANJIU

健 康 管 理 研 究

著　　者：	李凌姝　张　丽　徐　林　金光辉
出版策划：	崔文辉
责任编辑：	侯　帅
出　　版：	吉林出版集团股份有限公司
	（长春市福祉大路5788号，邮政编码：130118）
发　　行：	吉林出版集团译文图书经营有限公司
	（http://shop34896900.taobao.com）
电　　话：	总编办 0431-81629909　营销部 0431-81629880 / 81629900
印　　刷：	三河市金兆印刷装订有限公司
开　　本：	787mm×1092mm　1/16
印　　张：	19
字　　数：	400千字
版　　次：	2022年2月第1版
印　　次：	2023年6月第2次印刷
书　　号：	ISBN 978-7-5731-1126-5
定　　价：	48.00元

印装错误请与承印厂联系　电话：15901289808

前　言
PREFACE

　　健康管理（Health Management）一词起源于20世纪50年代的美国。随着时代的发展与人民生活水平的提高，健康管理的内容不断充实，相关研究也逐渐受到重视。从我国"十三五"规划提出的"大健康"建设，到《"健康中国2030"规划纲要》对我国医疗保障体系的发展与完善提出的新要求，无不表明全民健康管理水平的提高已被放在国家战略高度。与之相对的，则是被现代科技影响并改变的生活方式。在生活日渐便捷的同时，各种"懒人神器"的诞生让人们趋于懒惰；生活节奏的加快使竞争愈加激烈，过重的压力则会造成精神紧张，导致不良的生活习惯；这些因素都会导致不同程度的健康受损，从而成为疾病的诱因。

　　The term Health Management originated in the United States in the 1950s. With the development of the times and the improvement of people's living standards, the content of health management has been enriched and its related research is gradually gaining attention. From the "Great Health" proposed in China's 13th Five-Year Plan to the Outline of Healthy China 2030 Plan, which puts forward new requirements for the development of China's health care system, it is clearly shown that the improvement of nationwide health management has become a national strategy. In contrast, the way of life has been influenced and changed by modern technology. Life is increasingly convenient, but the appearance of various tools makes people become lazier. The acceleration of the pace of life makes competition more and more intense, while excessive pressure causes mental tension, which both lead to bad habits. These factors can all lead to different degrees of health impairment, which can be a trigger for diseases.

健康管理是一种对个人或人群的健康危险因素进行检测、分析、评估和干预的全面管理的过程，涉及社会、心理、环境、营养、运动等多个角度。良好的健康管理系统能够提供个性化的全面干预，大大降低疾病风险，从而提高健康水平和个体生活质量。然而，健康管理研究领域仍有较大缺口有待填补，该领域的学术研究远未达到成熟阶段。同时，由于健康管理在我国仍然属于新兴概念，有关健康管理的研究较少且认知度不高，健康管理的一些理念尚未被公众所接受。在此背景下，健康管理研究的展开显得尤为重要。

Health management is a comprehensive process of detecting, analysing, evaluating and intervening in the health risk factors of an individual or a group, involving various aspects such as society, psychology, environment, nutrition, sports and others. A good health management system provides individualized comprehensive interventions to significantly reduce the risk of disease, thus improving health and the quality of life. However, there are still large gaps to be filled in the field of health management research. Academic research in this area is far from reaching a mature stage. At the same time, as health management is still a new concept in China, research in this field is scarce and has a low awareness. What's more, some of its ideas are not yet accepted by the public. In this context, the development of health management research is particularly important.

本书内容丰富、结构严谨、逻辑清晰，注重章节间的紧密联系，不仅阐述了健康管理的基本概念、原则、理论及其趋势发展，更将专业知识带入生活中的具体情境，集系统性、科学性、实用性为一体。此外，本书通过中英双语对照的方式介绍相关研究，以期提升健康管理研究领域的国际视野，从而使读者在进一步理解和掌握理论知识的同时，对国内外的健康管理实践与研究建立相对全面的了解。健康管理是运用跨领域现代技术、聚焦现代健康需求的新兴概念,健康管理的研究必将随着时代进步而扩展充实,其学术领域中也仍有许多问题需要更深入的研究。

This book is informative, well-structured as well as logical, with an emphasis on a high degree of integration between chapters. It not only describes the basic concepts, principles, theories and trends of health management, but also combines professional knowledge with specific situations in reality, which integrates systematicness, scientificity and practicality. In addition, this book introduces relevant research in both Chinese and English in order to enhance the international perspective in the field of health management research. In this way, it can enable readers to have a relatively comprehensive understanding of the practice and research of health management at home and abroad while further understanding and mastering the theoretical knowledge. As health management's being an emerging concept that uses modern cross-disciplinary techniques and focuses on modern health needs, the study of health management is bound to expand and enrich with time. Also, there are still many issues in the academic field that require more in-depth research.

本书由李凌姝、张丽、徐林、金光辉共同撰写完成,具体分工如下:

This book is co-authored by Lingshu Li, Li Zhang, Lin Xu and Guanghui Jin, with the following division of labour:

李凌姝:第二章、第三章、第八章第一节(共计18万字);

张丽:第五章第一节至第四节、第七章、第八章第二节(共计9万字);

徐林:第一章、第六章(共计7万字);

金光辉:第四章、第五章第五节至第六节(共计6万字)。

Lingshu Li: Chapter Two, Chapter Three, Chapter Eight Section One(180,000 words in total)

Li Zhang: Chapter Five Section One to Four, Chapter Seven, Chapter Eight Section Two (90,000 words in)

Lin Xu: Chapter One, Chapter Six (70,000 words in total)

Guanghui Jin: Chapter Four, Chapter Five Section Five to Six (60,000 words in total)

最后，由李凌姝对全书进行了统稿与定稿。在此，感谢上海外国语大学教务处和体育教学部领导的大力支持。同时，复旦大学、上海外国语大学、湖南工业大学以及华东师范大学的学生朱立君、夏正选、叶晗清、江雨墨、管佳乐、冯思哲、曹雷、李艳、刘晨曦、王俊贤在本书撰写过程中做了大量的资料收集和文字处理与校对工作，正是他们的精诚合作和共同努力，保障了本书的品质。

At last, Lingshu Li unified and finalized this book. We would like to thank the leaders of the Academic Affairs Office and the Department of Physical Education of Shanghai International Studies University for their support. Meanwhile, Lijun Zhu, Zhengxuan Xia, Hanqing Ye, Yumo Jiang, Jiale Guan, Sizhe Feng, Lei Cao, Yan Li, Chenxi Liu, Junxian Wang from Fudan University, Shanghai International Studies University, Hunan University of Technology and East China Normal University did a great deal of data collection, word processing and proofreading work during the writing process of this book. It was their sincere cooperation and joint efforts that guaranteed the quality of this book.

本书在撰写过程中，参阅了众多文献，在此，谨向有关作者致以衷心的敬意与感谢。

本书虽然几经修改，但是限于作者水平有限，难免存在疏漏之处，殷切期望读者朋友提出宝贵意见和建议，同时期待专家同行批评指正！

In the course of writing this book, numerous references have been made. Here, I would like to express my sincere respect and gratitude to the authors concerned. Although this book has been revised several times, there are unavoidable omissions due to the author's limitations. So we earnestly hope that readers will make valuable comments and suggestions on it, and look forward to the criticism and correction of peer experts!

李凌姝

Lingshu Li

2021年10月7日于上海

(Shanghai, 7th Oct. 2021)

目 录
CONTENTS

第一章 健康管理概论 ··· 001
CHAPTER ONE GENERAL DESCRIPTION OF HEALTH MANAGEMENT

 第一节 健康及其重要性 ·· 002
 Section One Health and Its Importance

 第二节 健康管理简介 ·· 008
 Section Two Introduction to Health Management

 第三节 健康的影响因素与健康管理的基本策略 ············ 019
 Section Three Influencing Factors of Health and Basic Strategies of Health Management

 第四节 健康管理的实施途径 ································· 030
 Section Four Implementation of Health Management

第二章 体育锻炼、营养与健康 ································· 033
CHAPTER TWO EXERCISE, NUTRITION AND HEALTH

 第一节 体重控制 ·· 034
 Section One Weight Control

 第二节 营养与体能 ·· 051

Section Two Nutrition and Physical Agility

第三章　体育锻炼与心理、社会健康 ·········· 060
CHAPTER THREE EXERCISE AND MENTAL & SOCIAL HEALTH

第一节　体育锻炼与心理健康 ·········· 061

Section One Exercise and Mental Health

第二节　体育锻炼与社会健康 ·········· 075

Section Two Exercise and Social Health

第三节　体育锻炼与应激 ·········· 079

Section Three Exercise and Stress Control

第四章　健康管理基本操作技能 ·········· 092
CHAPTER FOUR BASIC OPERATION SKILLS OF HEALTH MANAGEMENT

第一节　简单的测量身体健康状况的操作 ·········· 093

Section One Operation and Measurement of Health Condition

第二节　身体活动水平的测量 ·········· 103

Section Two Measurement of Activity

第五章　健康教育与健康促进 ·········· 122
CHAPTER FIVE HEALTH EDUCATION AND HEALTH PROMOTION

第一节　健康行为 ·········· 122

Section One Health Behaviour

第二节　健康教育 ·········· 127

Section Two Health Education

第三节　健康促进 ·········· 135

Section Three Health Promotion

第四节　健康传播 ·· 139
Section Four Health Transmission

第五节　社区健康教育 ··· 142
Section Five Community Health Education

第六节　健康教育与健康促进的计划设计 ······················ 146
Section Six Planning for Health Education and Health Promotion

第六章　健康风险评估与风险管理 ···························· 159
CHAPTER SIX HEALTH RISK ASSESSMENT AND RISK MANAGEMENT

第一节　健康风险评估的相关概念与历史 ····················· 160
Section One Concept and History of Health Risk Assessment

第二节　健康风险评估的目的、应用和技术方法 ············· 165
Section Two Objectives, Applications and Technical Methods of Health Risk Assessment

第三节　健康风险评估的种类和注意事项 ····················· 172
Section Three Types and Considerations of Health Risk Assessment

第七章　健康保险与健康管理 ································· 182
CHAPTER SEVEN HEALTH INSURANCE AND HEALTH MANAGEMENT

第一节　健康保险概述 ··· 183
Section One Overview of Health Insurance

第二节　我国健康保险的现状和发展趋势 ····················· 195
Section Two Present Situation and Trends of Health Insurance in China

第三节　健康保险行业中健康管理的概述 ····················· 205
Section Three Overview of Health Management in Health Insurance Industry

第四节　健康保险与健康管理的关系 ……………………………………… 209

Section Four Relationship Between Health Insurance and Health Management

第五节　新时代健康保险的发展 …………………………………………… 214

Section Five Development of Health Insurance in the New Era

第八章　生活方式与健康管理 …………………………………………… 218

CHAPTER EIGHT LIFE STYLE AND HEALTH MANAGEMENT

第一节　慢性病患者的生活方式与健康管理 ……………………………… 219

Section One Lifestyle and Health Management of Chronic Disease Patients

第二节　运动方式与健康管理 ……………………………………………… 251

Section Two Exercise Mode and Health Management

参考文献 …………………………………………………………………… 287

REFERENCE

第一章 健康管理概论
CHAPTER ONE GENERAL DESCRIPTION OF HEALTH MANAGEMENT

随着社会不断发展和人民生活水平的提高,健康成为大众所日益关心的问题。而健康不仅是指身体健康,还包括心理健康、社会适应良好和道德健康。21世纪是更加注重健康管理的新时代,我们需要对健康以及健康管理具有一个良好的认知观,才能更好地摆脱高血压、肥胖等现代病。本章将从健康管理的定义、内容、发展史和基本特点等方面着手,帮助大家在了解健康管理的同时,树立一个良好的健康观。

With the continuous development of society and improvement of people's living standards, health has become an increasingly concern for the public. Health not only refers to physical health, but also includes mental health, social wellbeing and moral health. The 21st century is a new era in which people pay more attention to health management. We should have a good perception of health and health management in order to prevent modern diseases such as hypertension and obesity. This chapter will explain the definition, content, history and characteristics of health management to help people understand health management and set up a good view of health.

第一节 健康及其重要性
Section One Health and Its Importance

一、健康的定义
Definition of Health

根据世界卫生组织给出的健康定义，健康不仅指没有疾病，而且包括躯体健康、心理健康、社会适应良好和道德健康。

According to the definition of health given by the World Health Organization, health is a state of complete physical, mental, social wellbeing and moral health, and not merely the absence of disease.

二、我国社会目前面临的健康问题
Health Problems in China

（一）癌症
Cancer

癌症被认为是导致病人死亡最多的一种疾病。据国家癌症中心统计，全球每年新发癌症病例1400多万，我国每年新发病例429万。肺癌是我国发生率和死亡率最高的癌症，过去30年间死亡率上升了465%。

Cancer is considered to be the disease that kills the most patients. According to the statistics of the National Cancer Center, there are more than 14 million new cancer cases worldwide every year, and 4.29 million new cancer cases in China every year. Lung cancer is the most prevalent and deadliest cancer in our country, with a 465% increase in mortality over the past 30 years.

（二）慢性病
Chronic Diseases

近年来，以心血管疾病、糖尿病、慢性阻塞性肺病和恶性肿瘤为代表的慢性疾病已经成为我国的头号健康杀手。2018年，我国首部健康管理蓝皮书《中国健康管理与健康产业发展报告》发布。蓝皮书指出，我国慢性病发病人数在3亿左右，其中65岁以下人群慢性病负担占50%。我国城市和农村因慢性病死亡占总死亡人数的比例分别高达85.3%和79.5%。

In recent years, chronic diseases, represented by cardiovascular disease, diabetes, chronic obstructive pulmonary disease and malignant tumor, have done most harm to health in China. In 2018, China's first blue book of health management *Annual Report on Development of Health Management and Health Industry in China* was released. It pointed out that the number of people suffering from chronic diseases in China is about 300 million, with the burden of chronic diseases among people under 65 years of age accounting for 50%. In China, the proportion of deaths due to chronic diseases in China's urban and rural areas was as high as 85.3% and 79.5% of the total number of deaths respectively.

（三）心理疾病和肥胖

Mental Illness and Obesity

据世界卫生组织统计，中国有心理问题的人数达到2亿～3亿，每年约有28.7万人自杀，200万人企图自杀。肥胖问题也常常被人们所忽视，数据显示在中国有27.8%的成年人超重，我国的肥胖人口比例约为5.5%。肥胖能够带来一系列健康问题，如心血管疾病、心理与社会问题等。

According to the World Health Organization, 200-300 million people in China have psychological problems, with about 287 thousand people commit suicide every year, and 2 million people attempt to commit suicide. Obesity is also often ignored by people. The data shows that 27.8% of adults in China are overweight, and the proportion of obese population in China is about 5.5%. Obesity can bring a series of health problems, such as cardiovascular disease, psychological and social problems and so on.

三、名人的健康问题

Health Problems of Celebrities

（一）苹果公司的创始人史蒂夫·乔布斯

Steve Jobs, the Founder of Apple

2003年10月，48岁的乔布斯被确诊为胰腺癌，分别在2004年7月、2009年接受了治疗和手术，8年之后由于体内胰腺肿瘤转移后导致呼吸骤停去世。

In October 2003, Jobs was diagnosed with pancreatic cancer at 48 years old. He received treatment and surgery in July 2004 and 2009 respectively. Eight years later, he died of respiratory arrest due to metastasis of pancreatic tumor.

（二）著名的央视主持人李咏

Li Yong, a Famous CCTV Host

李咏患癌症在美国接受了17个月的治疗后，在2018年10月25日去世，时年50岁。

After 17 months of treatment in the United States for cancer, Li Yong died on October 25, 2018 at the age of 50.

（三）中央电视台著名播音员罗京

Luo Jing, a Famous Broadcaster of CCTV

罗京于2008年奥运前夕检查出淋巴癌，2009年6月5日去世。

Luo Jing was diagnosed with lymphatic cancer on the eve of the 2008 Olympic Games and died on June 5, 2009.

四、中国在健康领域面临的挑战

Challenges faced by China in the field of health

（一）传染病与非传染病的双重威胁

Dual Threat of Infectious and Non-Infectious Diseases

1. HIV感染人数迅速增加

Number of People Infected with HIV Increases Rapidly

在2012年12月，全国报告存活HIV感染者共24万人，截至2019年10月底，全国报告存活感染者95.8万，相较于2012年已然翻了两番。而2019年全年新发现感染者（根据2019年1—10月疫情数据预测），相较于2012年，也将翻一番。HIV疫情扩散增速平稳，新发现HIV感染者以每年1万人的速度加速增长。

In December 2012, a total of 240,000 people were reported to be living with HIV nationwide. By the end of October 2019, 958,000 people were reported to be living with HIV nationwide, which has quadrupled compared with 2012. The number of newly found infections in 2019 (according to the forecast of epidemic data from January to October 2019) will double compared with 2012. The speed of spread of HIV epidemic is growing steadily, and the number of newly found HIV infected people is accelerating at an annual rate of 10000.

2. 肺结核患者数量居世界第二

The Amount of Tuberculosis Patients Rank Second in the World

结核病是一种经呼吸道传播的慢性传染病，是我国重点控制的重大疾病之一。我国结核病患者数量居世界第二位，其中75%在农村，目前有结核菌感染者5.5亿人，结核病患者500万人，每年死于结核病的约13万人。

Tuberculosis(TB) is a chronic infectious disease transmitted by respiratory tract, which is one of the major diseases that China is focusing on and controlling. The number of TB patients in China ranks second in the world, 75% of which are in rural areas. Currently, there are 550 million TB-infected people, 5 million TB patients, and about 130000 people die of TB every year.

3. 乙肝病毒携带者占世界的近1/3

Hepatitis B Virus Carriers Account for Nearly One Third of the World

全球乙肝病毒携带者约有3.5亿人，其中中国有近1亿人。该病常无症状表现，但日后可发展为肝硬化或肝癌。

There are about 350 million hepatitis B virus carriers in the world, of which nearly 100 million are in China. The disease is often asymptomatic, but it can later develop into cirrhosis of the liver or liver cancer.

4. 新发传染病威胁严重

Serious Threats of Emerging Infectious Diseases

近年来，严重急性呼吸道症候群、新型冠状病毒性肺炎等严重威胁人类健康与生命。

In recent years, severe acute respiratory syndrome (SARS) and coronavirus pneumonia have become serious threats to human health and life.

（二）未富先老，未老先衰

Getting Old before Getting Rich, Getting Old before One's Time

1999年中国有老年人1.26亿，呈现出10%老龄化的形式，亚洲有老年人3.14亿，全世界共5.93亿。预计到2050年中国老龄化将会上涨到30%，老龄化人口基数将达到4.1亿，城乡居住比例为城镇34%，农村66%。

In 1999, there were 126 million elderly people in China, showing a form of aging of 10% while there were 314 million elderly people in Asia, and a total of 593 million worldwide. It is estimated that by 2050, China's aging population will rise to 30%, and the aging population base will reach 410 million. The proportion of urban and rural residents will be 34% in urban areas and 66% in rural areas.

（三）人口基数大，性别比失衡

The Large Population Base and the Imbalanced Sex Ratio

截至2018年，我国内地总人口约为14亿人（不包括港澳台同胞），中国的男女比例是116.9∶100，男性比女性多3000万～4000万。我国男女比例一直不平衡，不过目前已经逐渐好转。

As of 2018, the total population of Chinese mainland is about 14 billion (not including Chinese in Hong Kong, Macao and Taiwan). The ratio of men to women in China is 116.9:100, with 30 to 40 million more men than women. The proportion of men and women is always imbalanced, but the situation has gradually been improved.

五、我国在健康领域新的挑战

New Challenges in the Field of Health in China

（一）城镇化是新世纪对中国的一大挑战

Urbanization Is a Great Challenge to China in the New Century

近3亿农村人口向城市人口转化导致人口流动和城市人口密集，住房和交通拥挤，生活空间缩小，工作压力增加，为传染病流行提供了很好的条件。

The transformation of nearly 300 million rural population into urban population has led to population mobility and urban population density, housing and traffic congestion, shrinking living space and increasing work pressure, which provide good conditions for the epidemic of infectious diseases.

（二）城镇化和全球化带来了现代病——肥胖

Urbanization and Globalization Bring Modern Disease-Obesity

儿童肥胖导致运动障碍、肝脂肪变性、高血压、胆石症以及治疗费用逐年增加。

Obesity in children leads to dyskinesia, hepatic steatosis, hypertension, cholelithiasis and the increasing cost of treatment.

（三）我国人口学特征的变化

Changes of Demographic Characteristics in China

步入老龄化社会，慢性疾病患病率迅速上升，慢性病相关危险因素的流行日益严重，医疗费用急剧上涨，个人、集体和政府不堪重负。

As we enter an aging society, the prevalence of chronic diseases is rising rapidly, the prevalence of risk factors associated with chronic diseases is growing, and the cost of healthcare is rising sharply, overwhelming individuals, groups and governments.

（四）健康保障模式的变化

Changes of Health Insurance Mode

社会医疗保障下降，个人卫生支出增加，城镇化发展较快，肥胖率上升。

As social medical security declines, personal health expenditure increases. Meanwhile, urbanization has developed rapidly, and obesity rate has increased.

第二节 健康管理简介
Section Two Introduction to Health Management

一、健康管理的基本内容

Basic Content of Health Management

（一）定义

Definition

1. 管理

Management

管理是对个体或群体的健康进行全面监测、分析、评估、提供健康咨询和指导以及对健康危险因素进行干预的全过程，实质上是人们为了实现一定的目标而采取的手段，包括制定战略计划和目标、管理资源、使用完成目标所需要的人力和财务资本，以及衡量结果的组织过程。

Management is the whole process of comprehensive monitoring, analysis, evaluation, health consultation and guidance, and intervention in health risk factors for individuals or groups. In essence, it is a means that people take in order to achieve certain goals, including making strategic plans and goals, managing resources, using human and financial resources needed to achieve the goals and organizational process of evaluating results.

2. 健康管理

Health Management

广义上，随着实际业务内容的不断充实和发展，健康管理逐步发展成为一套专门的系统方案和营运业务，开始出现区别于医院等传统医疗机构的专业健康管理公司，作为第三方服务机构与医疗保险机构或直接面向个体需求，提供系统专业的健康管理服务。狭义的健康管理是指基于健康体检结果，建立专属健康档案，给出健康状况评估，并有针对性地提出个性化健康管理方案（处方），据此，由专业人士提供一对一咨询指导和跟踪辅导服务，使客户从社会、心理、环境、营养、运动等多个角度得到全面的健康维护和保障服务。

In a broad sense, with continuous enrichment and development of actual business content, health management has gradually developed into a set of specialised system solutions and operation business. And professional health management companies, different from hospitals and other traditional medical institutions, begin to appear. They provide systematic and professional health management services as third-party service institutions and medical insurance institutions, or directly base on individual needs. In a narrow sense, health management refers to establishment of an exclusive health file based on results of health check-ups, giving an assessment of health conditions and proposing a personalized health management plan (prescription), based on which professionals provide one-to-one advisory guidance and follow-up counselling services. In this way, customers can receive comprehensive health maintenance and security services from the perspectives of society, psychology, environment, nutrition, sports and so on.

（二）宗旨与特点

Purposes and Characteristics

1. 健康管理的宗旨

Purposes of Health Management

调动个体和群体及整个社会的积极性，有效地利用有限的资源来达到最大的健康效果。健康管理一般不涉及疾病的诊断和治疗过程，是一种对个人或人群的健康危险因素进行检测、分析、评估和干预的全面管理的过程。

Mobilizing individuals and groups, as well as the whole society, can be an effective way of using limited resources to achieve maximum health outcomes. Health management generally does not involve the process of disease diagnosis and treatment; it is a comprehensive management process to detect, analyze, evaluate and intervene in health risk factors for individuals or groups.

2. 健康管理的特点

Characteristics of Health Management

（1）以控制健康危险因素为核心

Health Management Focuses on Controlling Health Risk Factors

健康管理以控制健康危险因素为核心，包括可变危险因素和不可变危险因素。前者为通过自我行为改变的可控因素，如不合理饮食、缺乏运动、吸烟酗酒等不良生活方式，高血压、高血糖、高血脂等异常指标因素。后者为不受个人控制因素，如年龄、性别、家族史等因素。

Health management focuses on controlling health risk factors, including variable and immutable ones. The former are controllable factors that can be changed through self-monitoring, such as unreasonable diet, lack of exercise, smoking and drinking, hypertension, hyperglycemia, hyperlipidemia and other abnormal index factors. The latter is not controlled by individuals, such as age, gender, family history and so on.

（2）具有三级预防

Health Management Has Three Levels of Prevention

健康管理具有三级预防：①无病预防，又称病因预防，是在疾病尚未发生时针对病因或危险因素采取措施，降低有害暴露的水平，增强个体对抗有害暴露的能力，预防疾病的发生或至少推迟疾病的发生。②临床前期预防，即疾病早发现早治疗。在疾病的临床前期做好早期发现、早期诊断、早期治疗的"三早"预防措施。这一级的预防是通过早期发现、早期诊断而进行适当的治疗，来防止疾病临床前期或临床初期的变化，能使疾病在早期就被发现和治疗，避免或减少并发症、后遗症和残疾的发生，或缩短致残的时间。③治病防残，又称临床预防。三级预防可以防止伤残和促进功能恢复，提高生存质量，延长寿命，降低病死率。

Health management has three levels of prevention. ①Disease-free prevention, also known as etiological prevention, is to take measures to reduce the level of harmful exposure, enhance the ability of individuals to resist harmful exposure, prevent the occurrence of disease or at least delay the occurrence of disease. ②Preclinical prevention means early detection and early treatment. In the early clinical stage of the disease, we should take the "three-early" preventive measures, which refer to early detection, early diagnosis and early treatment. This level of prevention is to prevent the changes of the disease in preclinical or early clinical stage through early detection, early diagnosis and appropriate treatment, so that the disease can be found and treated at an early stage, the occurrence of complications, sequelae and disability can be avoided or redwced, and the time of disability can be shorten. ③Treatment and prevention of disability is also known as clinical prevention. Tertiary prevention can prevent disability is promote functional recovery, improve quality of life, prolong life span and reduce mortality.

（3）健康管理的服务过程为环形运转循环

Service Process of Health Management Is a Circular Operation Cycle

健康管理的服务过程为环形运转循环，实施环节为健康监测、健康评估、健康干预。整个服务过程，通过这三个环节不断循环运行，可以减少或降低危险因素的个数和级别，保持低风险水平。

Service process of health management is a circular operation cycle, and the implementation links are health monitoring, health assessment and health intervention. The entire service process, operating in a continuous cycle through these three components, is able to reduce or lower the number and level of risk factors and maintain a low level of risk.

二、健康管理的起源与发展

Origin and Development of Health Management

（一）健康管理的起源

Origin of Health Management

1. 中国古代健康管理的起源

Origin of Health Management in Ancient China

中国古代健康管理思想的雏形起源于《黄帝内经》——"上医治未病，中医治欲病，下医治已病"，即医术最高明的医生并不是擅长治病的人，而是能够预防疾病的人。

The rudiment of ancient Chinese health management thought originated from *Huangdi Neijing*, which claimed that the most skillful doctors are not only good at treating diseases, but also prevent diseases.

2. 西方古代健康管理的起源

Origin of Ancient Western Health Management

西方古代健康管理思想的雏形起源于希波克拉底思想，他是古希腊伯里克利的医师，被西方尊为"医学之父"、西方医学奠基人。他认为抵制疾病是神赐予的谬说，并且长期努力探究人的肌体特征和疾病的成因。经过长期的努力，他提出了体液学说，认为人体由血液、黏液、黄疸和黑胆四种体液组成，这四种体液的不同配合使人们有不同的体质。他把疾病看作是发展着的现象，认为医师所应医治的不仅是病而是病人，从而改变了当时医学中以巫术和宗教为根据的观念。

The rudiment of ancient Western health management thought originated from Hippocratic thoughts. He was a doctor of Pericles in ancient Greece, respectfully known as "Father of Medicine" and the founder of Western medicine. He believed that resisting disease is a god given fallacy, and devoted himself to exploring characteristics of human body and causes of disease. By sustained efforts, he put forward the theory of body fluid, which claimed that the human body was composed of four body fluids: blood, phlegm, yellow bile and black bile. Different combinations of these four body fluids brought people different constitutions. He regarded disease as a developing phenomenon, and believed that what doctors should treat was not only the disease but the patient, which changed the concept of medicine based on witchcraft and religion at that time.

3. 现代健康管理的起源

Origin of Managed Care

现代健康管理（Managed Care）是20世纪50年代末最先在美国提出的概念，当时被称作医疗保健，它的目的是加强健康管理和疾病控制的有效性，以减少公众的医疗费用。其核心内容是医疗保险机构通过对其医疗保险客户（包括疾病患者或高危人群）开展系统的健康管理，达到有效控制疾病的发生或发展，显著降低出险概率和实际医疗支出，从而减少医疗保险赔付损失的目的。1948年，美国总统杜鲁门向全体美国国民发布第一部健康白皮书《告美国人民健康白皮书》，指出美国人民面临严峻的健康问题，引起全民健康思考，现代健康管理萌芽产生。美国经过20多年的研究得出了这样一个结论，即任何企业及个人都有这样一个秘密，即所谓的90%和10%：90%的个人和企业通过健康管理后，医疗费用降到原来的10%；10%的个人和企业没有进行健康管理，医疗费用比原来上升90%。随后，健康管理观念传入欧洲，并逐步扩展到全世界范围。我国在"十三五"规划之后，提出了"大健康"建设的概念，将国民健康管理提升到国家战略层面。根据"规划"，群众健康管理将从医疗转向预防为主，不断提高民众的自我健康管理意识。

  Modern Heath Management is a concept first developed in the United States in the late 1950s. At that time, known as health care, it aimed to enhance the effectiveness of health management and disease control in order to reduce the cost of healthcare to the public. The core is promoting systematic health management of health insurance clients, including those with illnesses or at risk, to effectively control the occurrence or progression of illnesses and significantly reduce the probability of risk and actual medical expenses, thereby reducing the loss of health insurance benefits. In 1948, US President Harry S. Truman issued the first white paper on health, *"White Paper on the Health of American People"* to all American citizens, pointing out the serious health problems faced by American people, causing all people to think about health and the emergence of modern health management. After more than 20 years of research, the United States concluded that health management had such a secret for any enterprise and individual, that is, 90% and 10%. After 90% of individuals and enterprises achieved health management, the medical expenses would drop to 10% of the original; 10% of individuals and enterprises do not carry out health management, and the medical expenses will rise by 90%. Subsequently, the concept of health management was introduced into Europe and gradually extended to the whole world. After the 13th Five-Year Plan, China puts forward the concept of "Great Health" construction, which promoted national health management to the national strategic level. According to the "plan", people's health management will shift from medical treatment to prevention, and the state strives to improve people's awareness of self-health management.

（二）我国健康管理的发展

Development of Health Management in China

健康管理在我国的发展至今已有20多年，理论研究也相对空白，但已经有了各类实践与应用。2001年我国第一家健康管理公司正式注册成立，2004年，中国保监会批准的中国第一家专业健康保险公司成立。2005年，中国劳动和社会保障部正式向社会发布了第四批11个新职业，包括健康管理师，有力地推动了健康管理在我国的发展。2007年，《健康管理师国家管理标准》正式公布。2008年，我国正式提出"健康中国2020"战略，针对健康问题和影响健康的危险因素，积极采取经济有效的干预措施和适当的卫生策略，努力提高全民健康水平。2009年，卫生部出台《健康体检管理暂行规定》。在之后的十年间，我国出台了健康管理的报告和条例，并采取积极措施改善公共卫生。2018年，我国发布首部《健康管理蓝皮书：中国健康管理与健康产业发展报告》。

Health management has been developing in China for more than 20 years till now and the theoretical research is relatively blank, but there have been various kinds of practice and application. In 2001, China's first health management company was officially registered. In 2004, China's first professional health insurance company approved by CIRC was established. In 2005, China's Ministry of Labor and Social Security officially released the fourth batch of 11 new occupations, including health managers, which effectively promoted the development of health management in China. In 2007, the national management standard for health administrators was officially published. In 2008, China formally put forward the "Healthy China 2020" strategy, aiming at health problems and risk factors affecting health, by actively taking economic and effective intervention measures and appropriate health strategies, and strived to improve the health level of the whole people. In 2009, the Ministry of Health issued the Interim Provisions on the management of physical examination. In the following decade, China issued health management reports and regulations, and took positive measures to improve public health. In 2018, China released the first blue book of health management *Annual Report on Development of Health Management and Health Industry in China*.

三、健康管理的实施意义
Implementation Significance of Health Management

健康管理的目的在于使病人以及健康人群更好地恢复健康、维护健康、促进健康，并节约经费开支，有效降低医疗支出。大量预防医学研究表明，每在预防上花1元钱，就可以节省8.59元的医药费，还能相应节省约100元的抢救费、误工损失、陪护费等。社会各界人士都应该进行个人健康管理。

The purpose of health management is to make patients and healthy people better recover, maintain and promote health, save money and reduce medical expenses. A large number of preventive medicine studies have shown that every 1 yuan spent on prevention can save 8.59 yuan of medical expenses, and also save about 100 yuan of rescue costs, loss of work delay, accompanying costs, etc. People from all walks of life should carry out personal health management.

（一）健康人群
Healthy People

通过定期的健康评估来降低潜在的疾病风险。

Reduce the potential risk of disease through regular health assessment.

（二）亚健康人群
Sub-healthy People

通过科学的方法来达到健康。

Improve health through scientific methods.

（三）病人
Patients

通过健康管理，以健康跟踪的方式加以适当的治疗，来减轻或治愈疾病。

Through health management and appropriate treatment in the way of health tracking, the disease can be alleviated or cured.

四、健康管理的基本步骤和常用服务流程

Basic Steps and Common Service Process of Health Management

（一）基本步骤

Basic Steps

1. 了解你的健康

Know Your Health

了解自身的身体状况，包括身高、体重、有无过敏疾病史等。

Understand self-physical condition, including height, weight, history of allergic diseases and so on.

2. 进行健康与疾病的风险性评估

Conduct Health and Disease Risk Assessment

健康与疾病风险评估是健康管理过程中的关键部分，只有通过健康管理才能实现，是慢性病预防的第一步，也称为危险预测模型。收集个人健康信息，分析建立生活方式、环境、遗传等危险因素与健康状态之间的量化关系，预测个人在一定时间内发生某种特定疾病或因为某种特定疾病导致死亡的可能性，并据此按人群的需求提供有针对性的控制与干预，以帮助政府、企业、保险公司和个人，用最少的成本达到最大的健康管理效果。

Health and disease risk assessment is a key and irreplaceable part in the process of health management. It is the first step of chronic disease prevention, also known as risk prediction model. Collect personal health information, analyze and establish the quantitative relationship between lifestyle, environment, genetic and other risk factors and health status, predict the possibility of a specific disease or death caused by a specific disease within a certain period of time, then provide targeted control and intervention according to the needs of the population, so as to help the government, enterprises, insurance companies and individuals achieve the maximum health management effect with the least cost.

3. 进行健康干预
Health Intervention

健康干预为个体和群体（包括政府）提供有针对性的科学健康信息并创造条件采取行动来改善健康。

Health intervention provides targeted scientific health information for individuals and groups (including the government) and creates conditions for improving health.

（二）服务流程
Service Process

1. 健康管理体检
Health Management Physical Examination

健康管理体检是以健康为中心的身体检查，方便了解身体情况，筛查身体疾病。

Health management check-ups are health-focused physical examinations that facilitate understanding of the body and screening for physical illness.

2. 健康评估
Health Assessment

经过体检后的信息，由专业人士进行评估。

The information after physical examination is evaluated by professionals.

3. 个人健康咨询
Personal Health Consultation

个人健康咨询是通过询问健康管理过程中遇到的问题，以及可能发生的情况，进行专业性疏导。

Personal health consultation is to conduct professional counseling by asking about the problems encountered in the process of health management and the possible situations.

4. 个人健康管理服务
Personal Health Management Services

个人健康管理是根据个人生活习惯、个人病史、个人健康体检等方面的数据分析提供健康教育、健康评估、健康促进、健康追踪、健康督导和导医陪诊等专业化健康管理服务。个人因健康程度不同需要接受不同的健康管理服务。

Personal health management is to provide professional health management services such as health education, health assessment, health promotion, health tracking, health supervision and medical guidance according to the data analysis of personal living habits, personal medical history and personal health examination. Individuals will receive different health management services based on their different health levels.

（1）健康人群

Healthy People

热爱健康生活的群体已认识到健康的重要性，但由于健康知识不足，希望得到科学的、专业的、系统的、个性化的健康指导，并拟通过定期健康评估，保持在低风险水平，尽享健康人生。对于健康人群主要采取预防性健康管理（预防性服务、健康改善、受保人群的教育等）。

People who love a healthy lifestyle and have realized the importance of health, but due to lack of health knowledge, hope to get scientific, professional, systematic and personalized health guidance. And they plan to maintain a low level of health risk and enjoy a healthy life through regular health assessment. Preventive health management like preventive service, health improvement, education of insured people, etc. is mainly adopted for healthy people.

（2）亚健康人群

Sub-healthy People

亚健康人群指有四肢无力、心力交瘁、睡眠不好等症状的人群。由于从事的行业不同、社会竞争以及家庭负担的压力，他们明白自身处于亚健康状态但不知道如何改善，强烈要求采取措施提高工作效率和整体健康水平。

Sub-healthy people are those who suffer from weakness of limbs, mental and physical exhaustion, poor sleep and other. Due to different industries, social competition and family burden, people know they are in the sub-health state, but they do not know how to improve, so they strongly request to take measures to improve work efficiency and overall health level.

（3）疾病人群

Patients

疾病人群是在治疗的同时希望积极进行自身健康改善的群体。需要在临床治疗过程中在生活环境和行为方面进行全面改善，从而监控危险因素，降低风险水平，延缓疾病的进程，提高生命质量。对于一般疾病人群主要采取常规的医疗服务需求管理，不同慢性病、重病患者则采取不同的管理办法。

Patients are those who want to actively participate in their own health improvement at the same time of receiving treatment. In order to monitor risk factors, reduce the risk level, delay the process of disease and improve the quality of life, they need to improve the living environment and behavior in the process of clinical treatment. For people with general diseases, they mainly adopt conventional medical management, while different patients of chronic diseases and serious illness adopt different management.

第三节　健康的影响因素与健康管理的基本策略
Section Three Influencing Factors of Health and Basic Strategies of Health Management

一、影响人类健康的因素
Factors Affecting Human Health

（一）环境因素

Environmental Factor

环境因素包括自然环境、心理环境和社会环境。

Environmental factors include natural environment, psychological environment and social environment.

（二）生活方式及行为因素

Lifestyle and Behavioral Factors

生活方式是人们在社会化的过程中，在人们的相互影响下逐渐形成的。

Lifestyle is formed in the process of socialization and under the mutual influence of people.

（三）生物遗传因素

Biological Genetic Factors

生物遗传因素是理解生命活动和疾病的基础。

Biological genetic factors are the basis of understanding life activities and diseases.

（四）医疗卫生服务因素

Medical and Health Service Factors

医疗卫生服务是一种控制疾病的社会措施，医疗卫生服务的布局、资源的分配、卫生工作的方针、技术水平和服务质量是否符合人们的最大健康利益，都对人们的健康质量有着直接的影响。

Medical and health services are a social measure to control diseases. Whether layout of medical and health services, allocation of resources, policy of health work, technical level and quality of services are in line with people's best health interests has a direct impact on people's health quality.

二、健康管理基本策略的分类

Classification of Basic Health Management Strategies

（一）生活方式管理

Lifestyle Management

1. 定义与目的

Definition and Purpose

生活方式管理，从卫生服务的角度是指以个人为核心的卫生保健活动。该定义强调个人选择行为方式的重要性，因为其直接影响人们的健康。生活方式管理通过健康促进技术，比如行为纠正和健康教育，来保护人们远离不良行为，减少健康危险因素对健康的损害，预防疾病，改善健康。膳食、体力活动、吸烟、适度饮酒、精神压力等是目前国人生活方式管理的重点。

Lifestyle management, from the perspective of health services, refers to the health care activities centered on the individual. The definition emphasizes the importance of individual choice behavior, which directly affects people's health. Through health promotion technology, such as behavior correction and health education, lifestyle management can protect people from bad behaviors, reduce the damage of health risk factors to health, prevent diseases and improve health. Diet, physical activity, smoking, moderate drinking and mental stress are the key points of lifestyle management for Chinese people.

2. 特点

Characteristics

（1）以个体为中心，强调个体对自己的健康负责，调动个体的积极性，帮助个体做出最佳的健康行为

Taking the individual as the center, it emphasizes that the individual is responsible for his own health, mobilizing the individual's enthusiasm, and it helps the individual to perform the best health behavior

像不吸烟、不应挑食等都是人们应当坚持的生活方式，并且有利于健康生活，选择什么样的生活方式由个人的意愿或者行为所决定。通过提供条件供大家进行健康生活方式的体验，指导人们掌握改善生活方式的技巧这些渠道，可以帮助人们做出正确的决策，但这一切都不能替代个人做出选择何种生活方式的决策，即使一时替代性地做出，也很难长久坚持。

No smoking and no picky eating are lifestyles that people should adhere to, and it is conducive to the promotion of a healthy life. What kind of lifestyle you choose depends on your will or behavior. By providing conditions for people to experience healthy lifestyle and guiding people to master the skills of improving lifestyle, these channels can help people make correct decisions, but none of these can replace the individual's decision to choose a lifestyle; even if it is made for a while, it is difficult to stick to it for a long time.

（2）以预防为主，生活方式管理帮助个体改变行为，降低健康风险，促进健康，预防疾病和伤害，有效整合三级预防

Focusing on prevention, lifestyle management helps individuals change behaviors, reduce health risks, promote health, prevent diseases and injuries, and effectively integrate three-level prevention

预防是生活方式管理的核心，其含义不仅仅是预防疾病的发生，还在于逆转或延缓疾病的发展历程（如果疾病已不可避免的话）。因此，旨在控制健康危险因素，将疾病控制在尚未发生之时的一级预防；通过早发现、早诊断、早治疗而防止或减缓疾病发展的二级预防；以及防止伤残，促进功能恢复，提高生存质量，延长寿命，降低病死率的三级预防，在生活方式管理中都很重要，其中尤以一级预防最为重要。针对个体和群体的特点，有效地整合三级预防，而非孤立地采用三个级别的预防措施，是生活方式管理的真谛。

Prevention is the core of lifestyle management, which means not only to prevent the occurrence of diseases, but also to reverse or delay the development of diseases (if diseases are inevitable). Therefore, it is very important in lifestyle management to control health risk factors, control disease in the primary prevention before it occurs, prevent or slow down the development of disease through early detection, early diagnosis and early treatment, and prevent disability, promote functional recovery, improve quality of life, prolong life and reduce mortality. Among them, the primary prevention is the most important. According to the characteristics of individuals and groups, the essence of lifestyle management is to effectively integrate three levels of prevention, rather than to adopt three levels of prevention measures piecemeal.

（3）通常与其他健康管理策略联合进行

Usually in combination with other health management strategies

与许多医疗保健措施需要付出高昂费用为代价相反，预防措施通常是便宜而有效的，它们节约了更多的成本，收获了更多的边际效益。

Contrary conducted to the high cost of many health care measures, preventive measures are usually cheap and effective. They save more costs and gain more marginal benefits.

3. 生活方式管理的方法

Methods of Lifestyle Management

生活方式管理是其他群体健康管理策略的基础成分，单独应用或联合应用各类方法，可以帮助人们朝着有利于健康的方向改变生活方式。生活方式管理可以以多种不同的形式出现，也可以融入健康管理的其他策略中去。四种主要方法常用于促进人们改变生活方式。

Lifestyle management is the basic component of other groups' health management strategies. Individual or combined application of various methods can help people change their lifestyle in the direction of health. Lifestyle management can appear in many different forms, and can also be integrated into other strategies of health management. Four main methods are commonly used to promote lifestyle change below.

（1）教育

Education

传递知识，确立态度，改变行为。

Impart knowledge, establish attitude and change behavior.

（2）激励

Encouragement

通过正面强化、反面强化、反馈促进、惩罚等措施进行行为矫正。

Correct behavior through positive reinforcement, negative reinforcement, feedback promotion, punishment and other measures.

（3）训练

Training

通过一系列的参与式训练与体验，培训个体掌握行为矫正的技术。

Master skills of behavior correction through a series of participatory training and experience.

（4）营销
Marketing

利用社会营销的技术推广健康行为，营造健康的大环境，促进个体改变不健康的行为。

Promote healthy behavior, create a healthy environment and promote individual change unhealthy behavior by social marketing technology.

（二）需求管理
Demand Management

1. 需求管理的概念
Concept of Demand Management

需求管理包括自我保健服务和人群就诊分流服务，帮助人们更好地使用医疗服务和管理自己的健康。实质上是通过帮助健康人士维护自身健康和寻求恰当的卫生服务，控制卫生成本，促进卫生服务的合理利用。

Demand management includes self-care service and triage service to help people better use medical services and manage their own health. In essence, it is to help healthy people maintain their own health and seek appropriate health services, control health costs and promote the rational use of health services.

2. 影响需求的因素
Factors Affecting Demand

（1）患病率
Prevalence

患病率可以影响卫生服务需求，它反映了人群中疾病的发生水平。但这并不表明患病率与服务利用率之间有良好的相关关系，相当多的疾病是可以预防的。

Prevalence can affect the demand for health services, which reflects the incidence of diseases in the population. However, this does not mean that there is a good correlation between the prevalence and service utilization. A considerable number of diseases are defendable.

(2) 感知到的需要
Perceived Needs

个人感知到的卫生服务需要是影响卫生服务利用的最重要的因素，它反映了个人对疾病重要性的看法，以及是否需要寻求卫生服务来处理该疾病。有很多因素影响着人们感知到的需要，包括：个人关于疾病危险和卫生服务益处的知识、个人评估疾病问题的能力、个人感知到的疾病的严重性、个人对自己处理好疾病问题的信心等。

The personal perceived need for health services is the most important factor affecting the utilization of health services. It reflects personal views on the importance of disease and whether it is necessary to seek health services to deal with the disease. There are many factors that affect people's perceived needs, including personal knowledge about disease risks and health service benefits, personal ability to assess disease problems, personal perceived severity of disease, personal confidence in dealing with disease problems.

(3) 病人偏好
Patient Preference

病人偏好的概念强调病人在决定其医疗保健措施时的重要作用。病人对选择何种治疗方法负责，医生的职责是帮病人了解这种治疗的益处和风险。

The concept of patient preference emphasizes the important role of patients in determining their health care measures. Patients are responsible for the choice of treatment, and doctors are responsible for helping patients understand the benefits and risks of such treatment.

(4) 健康因素以外的动机
Motivation Beyond Health Factors

一些健康因素以外的因素，如个人请病假的能力、疾病补助等都能影响人们寻求医疗保健的决定，保险中的自付比例也是影响卫生服务利用水平的一个重要因素。

Some factors other than health factors, such as personal ability to take sick leave, disease subsidies and so on, can affect people's decision to seek medical care. The out-of-pocket ratio in insurance is also an important factor affecting the utilization level of health services.

3. 需求预测方法与技术

Method and Technology of Demand Forecasting

（1）以问卷为基础的健康评估

Questionnaire-Based Health Assessment

以健康和疾病风险评估为代表，通过综合性的问卷和一定的评估技术，预测在未来的一定时间内个人的患病风险，以及谁将是卫生服务的主要消费者。

Taking health and disease risk assessment as the representative, through the comprehensive questionnaire and certain assessment technology, we can predict the individual disease risk in a certain period of time in the future, and who will be the main consumer of health services.

（2）以医疗卫生花费为基础的评估

Health Care Cost-Based Assessment

通过分析已发生的医疗卫生费用，预测未来的医疗花费。医疗花费数据是客观存在的，不会出现个人自报数据对预测结果的影响。

By analyzing medical and health costs already spent, we can predict future medical costs. The data of medical expenses is objective, and there is no influence of personal self-reported data on prediction results.

4. 需求管理的工具与实施策略

Tools and Implementation Strategies of Requirement Management

需求管理通常通过一系列的服务手段和工具影响和指导人们的卫生保健需求。常见的方法有：24小时电话就诊分流服务、转诊服务、基于互联网的卫生信息数据库、健康课堂、服务预约等。需求管理常用的实施策略包括：寻找手术的替代疗法、帮助病人减少特定的危险因素并采纳健康的生活方式、自我干预等。

Demand management usually influences and guides people's health care needs through a series of service means and tools. The common methods are: 24-hour telephone triage service, referral service, Internet-based health information database, health class, service appointment, etc. The common implementation strategies of demand management include: looking for alternative surgery, helping patients to reduce specific risk factors and adopt a healthy lifestyle, self intervention, etc.

（三）疾病管理

Disease Management

1. 定义

Definition

疾病管理是健康管理的又一主要策略，其历史发展较长。美国疾病管理协会对疾病管理的定义是：疾病管理是一个协调医疗保健干预和与病人沟通的系统，它强调病人自我保健的重要性。疾病管理支撑医患关系和保健计划，强调运用循证医学和增强个人能力的策略来预防疾病的恶化，它以持续性地改善个体或群体健康为基准来评估临床、人文和经济方面的效果。

Disease management is another major strategy of health management, which has a long history. Association of America (DMAA) defines disease management as a system to coordinate health care intervention and communication with patients, which emphasizes the importance of patients' self-care. Disease management supports doctor-patient relationship and health care plan, emphasizes the use of evidence-based medicine and strategy of enhancing individual ability to prevent the deterioration of disease, and evaluates the clinical, humanistic and economic effects based on the continuous improvement of individual or group health.

2. 特点

Characteristics

（1）目标人群是患有特定疾病的个体

The Target Population Is Individuals with Specific Diseases

如糖尿病管理项目的管理对象为已诊断患有Ⅰ型或Ⅱ型糖尿病的病人。

For example, the management object of diabetes management project is the patients who have been diagnosed with type Ⅰ or type Ⅱ diabetes.

（2）不以单个病例或其单次就诊事件为中心

Not Centered on a Single Case or Its Single Visit Event

该管理方法主要关注个体或群体连续性的健康状况与生活质量，这也是疾病管理与传统的单个病例管理的区别。

This management mainly focuses on the continuous health status and quality of life of individuals or groups, which is also the difference between disease management and traditional single case management.

（3）医疗卫生服务及干预措施的综合协调

Comprehensive Coordination of Medical and Health Services and Intervention Measures

疾病管理是一个协调医疗保健干预和与病人沟通的系统，它强调病人自我保健的重要性。

Disease management is a system of coordinating medical care intervention and communicating with patients, which emphasizes the importance of patients' self-care.

（四）灾难性病伤管理

Management of Catastrophic Diseases and Injuries

1. 定义

Definition

灾难性病伤管理是疾病管理的一个特殊类型，它关注的是"灾难性"的疾病或伤害。这里的"灾难性"可以是指对健康的危害十分严重，也可以是指其造成的医疗卫生花费巨大，常见于肿瘤、肾衰、严重外伤等情形。

Catastrophic disease and injury management is a special type of disease management, which focuses on "catastrophic" diseases or injuries. The "catastrophic" here can refer to the very serious harm to health, or the huge medical and health costs caused by it, which is common in tumor, renal failure, severe trauma and other situations.

2. 特点

Characteristics

灾难性病伤管理的特点包括：（1）转诊及时；（2）综合考虑各方面因素，制订出适宜的医疗服务计划；（3）具备一支包含多种医学专科及综合业务能力的服务队伍，能够有效应对可能出现的多种医疗服务需要；（4）最大限度地帮助病人进行自我管理；（5）患者及其家人满意。

The characteristics of catastrophic disease includes: (1) timely referral; (2) working out appropriate medical service plan after comprehensive consideration of various factors; (3) having a service team with multiple medical specialties and comprehensive professional abilities, which can effectively cope with the possible needs of various medical services; (4) helping patients to manage themselves to the greatest extent; (5) satisfying patients and their families.

（五）残疾管理

Disability Management

1. 定义

Definition

残疾管理是指通过预防和康复活动，使工伤和疾病所导致的健康损害可以得到及时的鉴定和治疗；残疾管理并不是对残疾人的护理，而是激发他们恢复健康并能够重新工作的动力。

Disability management refers to the timely identification and treatment of health damage caused by work-related injuries and diseases through prevention and rehabilitation activities. Disability management is not the care for the disabled, but the motivation to stimulate them to recover and work again.

2. 目的

Objective

残疾管理的目的在于减少工作地点发生残疾事故的频率和费用代价，防止残疾恶化，注重恢复功能性能力而不是减轻疼痛，设定实际康复和返工的期望值。

The purpose of disability management is to reduce the frequency and cost of disability accidents in the workplace, prevent the deterioration of disability, focus on recovering functional ability rather than alleviating pain, and set expectations for actual rehabilitation and rework.

（六）综合人群健康管理

Comprehensive Population Health Management

通过协调上述不同的健康管理策略来对个体提供更为全面的健康和福利

管理。这些策略都是以人的健康需要为中心而发展，健康管理实践中基本上应该都考虑采取综合的群体健康管理模式。

Coordinate the above different health management strategies, so as to provide more comprehensive health and welfare management for individuals. These strategies are all centered on people's health needs. And comprehensive group health management mode should be adopted in health management practice.

第四节　健康管理的实施途径
Section Four Implementation of Health Management

一、制定合理的管理政策，创设良好的锻炼环境
Formulate Reasonable Management Policies and Create a Good Exercise Environment

在健康管理创建和实施的过程中，科学的管理政策非常重要。此外，国家还应为不同阶层的人民提供一个良好的进行体育锻炼的氛围。政府在对管理政策进行制定的时候，需要对国家下发的相关文件有一个准确的认知和了解，然后完成对社会、学校、社区等地方管理文件的制定工作。在政策制定完成之后，政府还需要将其进行较好的落实。在对人民的健康进行管理的过程中，政府应该对各个部分所需要负责的内容进行明确划分，并安排一个部分专门用来对各个部门的工作情况及工作的质量进行监督，通过这个方式来有效保障政策更好地执行。

In the process of establishment and implementation of health management, it is very important to adopt scientific management policy. In addition, the state should provide a good atmosphere for people of different strata to do physical exercise. When the government formulates management policies, it needs to have an accurate understanding of the relevant documents issued by the state, and then complete the formulation of local management documents concerning society, schools and communities. After the completion of policy formulation, the government also needs to implement it accurately. In the process of the management of people's health, the government should clearly divide the contents of each part, and assign a part to supervise the work situation and quality of each department, so as to effectively guarantee the better implementation of policies.

二、科学健康健身指导

Scientific Health and Fitness Guidance

当前社会上存在的健身组织并不多，并且没有专门的部门进行管理，健身指导也有待提高，因而，政府部门应该要对相关的健身指导、健康管理政策进行完善，在不断的实践中发现不足，并且加以改进。

At present, there are not many fitness organizations in the society and there is no special department for management. Fitness guidance also needs to be improved as well. Therefore, the government should improve the relevant fitness guidance and health management policies, and find out the deficiencies in the continuous practice, and then improve them.

三、政府加大对体育设备资源的投入力度

Increase Investment in Sports Equipment by the Government

国家需增加对体育设备的资金投入量，对体育器材进行更换，并对操场等基础设施进行修补，从而让老百姓拥有一个良好的锻炼条件，这也有助于为老百姓提供良好的软硬件条件。

The state needs to increase the amount of investment in sports equipment, replace sports equipment, and repair the playground and other infrastructure, so that people have a good condition for exercise. In addition, it also helps to provide a good hardware and software conditions for the people.

思考

Questions

1. 健康管理是否会干涉医生的治疗计划？健康管理和医生的职责有什么不同？

Does health management interfere in doctors' treatment plans? What's the difference between the responsibilities of health management and doctors?

2. 举出一个健康管理的方案的例子，以说明健康管理中的一、二、三级预防。

Give an example of a health management program to illustrate the primary, secondary and tertiary prevention in health management.

第二章 体育锻炼、营养与健康
CHAPTER TWO EXERCISE, NUTRITION AND HEALTH

　　近年来，体育锻炼、营养与健康在我们的生活中变得愈加重要。越来越多的人开始注重体重控制，但太多的人使用了错误的方法，危害了自己的健康。同时，在营养搭配、体能训练方面，不少人走入了认识误区，以至于收效甚微。因此，本章将从体重控制、营养与体能两个方面入手，为保持健康体魄、拥有良好体能提供科学的介绍和建议。

　　In recent years, exercise, nutrition and health have become much more important in our lives. More and more people begin to pay attention to weight control, but too many people use the wrong method and therefore damage their health. At the same time, in terms of nutrition and physical training, many people have misunderstandings, so that they have little effect. Therefore, this chapter will start with two aspects of weight control, nutrition and physical fitness, and provide scientific introductions and suggestions for maintaining a healthy body and having good physical fitness.

第一节　体重控制
Section One Weight Control

一、肥胖与健康
Obesity and Health

（一）身体质量指数

Body Mass Index

1. 身体质量指数简介

Introduction of Body Mass Index

身体质量指数简称体质指数，通常也写作BMI指数（Body Mass Index），是目前国际上常用的衡量人体胖瘦程度以及是否健康的一个标准。当我们需要比较及分析一个人体的体重对于不同高度的人所带来的健康影响时，BMI值是一个中立而可靠的指标。

BMI值曾经是一个用于公众健康研究的统计工具。当时医学研究者需要知道肥胖是否为某一疾病的致病原因时，他们就可以将病人的身高体重换算作BMI值，再找出其数值是否与病发率存在线性关系。然而，随着科技的进步与更准确的度量方式（如体脂率、腰围身高比、内脏脂肪等）的出现，BMI指数也从医学统计工具变为一般大众的纤体指标。

The Body Mass Index is usually also written as the BMI index. It is a commonly used international standard to measure the degree of body weight and health. When we need to compare and analyze the health effects of a human body's weight on people of different heights, the BMI is a neutral and reliable indicator.

The BMI used to be a statistical tool for public health research. When the medical researchers need to know whether obesity is the cause of some certain diseases, they can convert the patient's height and weight into the body mass index, and then find out whether the value has a linear relationship with the incidence. However, with the advancement of technology and the emergence of more accurate measurement methods (such as body fat percentage, waist-to-height ratio, visceral fat, etc.), BMI has also changed from a medical statistical tool to a slimming indicator for the public.

2. BMI指数计算公式

Calculation Formula of BMI

BMI＝体重（千克）除以身高（米）的平方

BMI is calculated by dividing your body weight in kilograms by your height in meters squared.

身体质量指数适用于除孕妇和肌肉强健人群之外所有18至65岁的人群。由于不同人种体质上的差别，分为WHO和中国参考标准，可根据你的情况参照，自行评价。

BMI is suitable to all people between 18 and 65 years old except pregnant women and people with strong muscles. Due to the differences in physique of different races, it is divided into WHO and Chinese reference standards. You can follow the WHO or Chinese standards according to your own condition.

BMI指数的WHO标准、亚洲标准和中国参考标准对照表

BMI 分类	WHO标准	亚洲标准	中国参考标准
体重过低	BMI<18.5	BMI<18.5	BMI<18.5
正常范围	18.5≤BMI<25	18.5≤BMI<23	18.5≤BMI<24
超重	BMI≥25	BMI≥23	BMI≥24
肥胖前期	25≤BMI<30	23≤BMI<25	24≤BMI<28
Ⅰ度肥胖	30≤BMI<35	25≤BMI<30	28≤BMI<30
Ⅱ度肥胖	35≤BMI<40	30≤BMI<40	30≤BMI<40
Ⅲ度肥胖	BMI≥40.0	BMI≥40.0	BMI≥40.0

Comparison Table of WHO Standard, Asian Standard and Chinese Reference Standard of BMI

BMI Classification	WHO Standard	Asian Standard	Chinese Reference Standard
Underweight	BMI<18.5	BMI<18.5	BMI<18.5
Normal range	18.5≤BMI<25	18.5≤BMI<23	18.5≤BMI<24
Overweight	BMI≥25	BMI≥23	BMI≥24
Pre-obesity	25≤BMI<30	23≤BMI<25	24≤BMI<28
Obesity I	30≤BMI<35	25≤BMI<30	28≤BMI<30
Obesity II	35≤BMI<40	30≤BMI<40	30≤BMI<40
Obesity III	BMI≥40.0	BMI≥40.0	BMI≥40.0

（二）肥胖

Obesity

1. 肥胖的概念

Concept of Obesity

肥胖是指由于食物摄入过多或机体代谢的改变，而导致体内脂肪积聚过多，造成体重过度增长并引起人体病理、生理改变或潜伏。以体重指数对肥胖程度的分析，国际上通常用世界卫生组织（WHO）制定的体重指数界限值，即体重指数在25.0~29.9为超重，大于等于30为肥胖。国际生命科学学会中国办事处组织了由多学科专家组成的"中国肥胖问题工作组"，对我国21个省市、地区人群身体质量指数（BMI）、腰围、血压、血糖、血脂等24万人的相关数据进行汇总分析，并据此提出了中国人的BMI标准，BMI值"24"为中国成人超重的界限，BMI"28"为肥胖的界限；男性腰围≥85厘米，女性腰围≥80厘米为腹部脂肪蓄积的界限。由此可知，体重并不是判定肥胖的最准确指标，肥胖的实质是体内脂肪过多，而不是体重过高。

Obesity refers to excessive body fat accumulation due to excessive food intake or changes in body metabolism, which cause extra weight gain and pathological and physiological changes or certain potential risks to our health. We usually use the world-wide BMI standard established by the World Health Organization (WHO), that is, a body mass index of 25.0–29.9 is overweight, and a body mass index greater than or equal to 30 is obese. The China Office of the International Society of Life Sciences organized the "China Obesity Working Group" composed of multidisciplinary experts to assess the body mass index (BMI), waist circumference, blood pressure, blood sugar, and blood lipids of 240,000 people in 21 provinces, cities and regions in China. Relevant data is analyzed and the BMI standard for Chinese people is put forward. BMI "24" is the limit of Chinese adult overweight, BMI "28" is the limit of obesity; men's waist circumference ≥85 cm, women's waist circumference ≥ 80 cm are the limit of abdominal fat accumulation. It can be seen that weight is not the most accurate indicator of obesity. The essence of obesity is excess body fat, not excess weight.

2.常见的肥胖类型

Common Types of Obesity

本书介绍两种典型的肥胖类型，即苹果形肥胖和梨形肥胖。这两者间的区别在于脂肪在身体的不同部位的分布情况。目前判定正常、梨形和苹果形身材的方法包括测量腰围和测量腰围与臀围的比值，即腰臀比，可以和体格指数联合使用。腰围是反映脂肪总量和脂肪分布的综合指标，根据腰围检测肥胖症，很少发生错误。世界卫生组织推荐的测量方法是：被测者直立，双脚分开25～30厘米。测量者将皮尺放在最下面一根肋骨下缘与骨盆上缘（髂嵴）连线中点的水平位置进行测量。皮尺要紧贴着皮肤，但不能勒压软组织，测量应精确到0.1厘米。男性腰围大于90厘米即2尺7寸，女性腰围大于80厘米即2尺4寸，应视为苹果形肥胖。腰臀比的测定方法是：腰围÷臀围。其中臀围是水平测量臀部最宽部位的周径。如果男性的腰臀比值大于1，女性大于0.9，则为苹果形肥胖；如果男性小于0.8，女性小于0.7，则为梨形肥胖。

Here are two typical types of obesity, that is apple-shaped obesity and pear-shaped obesity. The difference between these two types lie in the distribution of fat in different parts of the body. The current methods for judging normal, pear-shaped and apple-shaped figures include measuring waist circumference and measuring the ratio of waist circumference to hip circumference, that is, waist-to-hip ratio, which can be used in conjunction with body mass index. Waist circumference is a comprehensive indicator that reflects the total amount of fat and fat distribution. Obesity can be measured by waist circumference and it rarely gets wrong. The measurement method recommended by the World Health Organization is: the subject stands upright with his feet 25-30cm apart. The tester places the measuring tape at the horizontal position of the midpoint of the line between the lower edge of the bottom rib and the upper edge of the pelvis (iliac crest) for measurement. The measuring tape should be close to the skin, but not the soft tissues. The measurement should be accurate to 0.1 cm. Men with a waist circumference greater than 90 cm are 2 feet 7 inches, and women with a waist circumference greater than 80 cm are 2 feet 4 inches, which should be regarded as apple-shaped obesity. The measurement of waist-hip ratio is to divide waist circumference by hip circumference. The hip circumference is a horizontal measurement of the circumference of the widest part of the buttocks. If the waist-to-hip ratio is greater than 1 for men and 0.9 for women, it is apple-shaped obesity; if it is less than 0.8 for men and 0.7 for women, it is pear-shaped obesity.

(1) 苹果形肥胖

Apple-shaped Obesity

苹果形肥胖患者的腰腹部过胖，状似苹果，细胳膊细腿大肚子，又称腹部型肥胖、向心型肥胖、男性型肥胖、内脏型肥胖，这种人脂肪主要沉积在腹部的皮下及腹腔内。

由于腹部脂肪比其他部位的脂肪新陈代谢更活跃，因此更易进入血液系统，可能导致高血压、高胆固醇及肥胖病。再有，苹果形肥胖患者的脂肪包围在心脏、肝脏、胰脏等重要器官周围，所以患冠心病、脂肪肝和糖尿病的危险性要比梨形肥胖大得多。有人发现肥胖者患糖尿病的危险性是普通人的3.7倍，而苹果形肥胖者患糖尿病的机会则高达不胖者的10.3倍。

The waist and abdomen of the apple-shaped body are overweight, which looks like an apple, with thin arms, thin legs and a big belly. They are also called abdominal obesity, centripetal obesity, male obesity, and visceral obesity. This kind of human fat is mainly deposited under the skin of the abdomen and in the abdominal cavity.

Because abdominal fat is more active than other parts of fat metabolism, it is easier to enter the blood system, which may cause high blood pressure, high cholesterol and obesity. In addition, the fat of apple-type obesity patients is surrounded by important organs such as the heart, liver, and pancreas, so the risk of coronary heart disease, fatty liver and diabetes is much greater than that of pear-type obesity. Some people have found that obese people are 3.7 times more likely to develop diabetes than ordinary people, while apple-shaped obese people have 10.3 times the risk of diabetes.

（2）梨形肥胖

Pear-shaped Obesity

梨形身材的人臀部及大腿脂肪过多，就是说脂肪主要沉积在臀部及大腿部，上半身不胖下半身胖，状似梨形。梨形肥胖的人群臀部也会出现大量的脂肪，并且也会出现下垂的问题。这类人群一般都比较喜欢吃甜食，除了正常的一日三餐以外，平时还喜欢吃零食和夜宵，而且饮食中所含的膳食纤维比较少。梨形身材一般出现在上班族，他们因为工作的原因需要长期久坐，这样就会出现臀部气血运行不畅的问题，从而导致腰间、臀部、大腿等多个部位囤积大量脂肪。如果平时有跷二郎腿的习惯，就会影响腿部的血液循环，从而导致下半身浮肿，并且出现脂肪不断增厚的问题，这样就会形成梨形身材。与非肥胖者相比，梨形肥胖仍然存在着相当严重的危险，仅仅是比苹果形肥胖略小而已。

People with a pear-shaped body have too much fat in the buttocks and thighs, which means that the fat is mainly deposited in the buttocks and thighs. The upper body is not fat and the lower body is fat, which looks like a pear shape. Pear-shaped obese people also have a lot of fat in their buttocks, which causes problems with sagging. Such people generally prefer to eat sweets. In addition to the normal three meals a day, they also like to eat snacks and extra meal at night, and their diet contains less dietary fiber. Pear-shaped figures generally appear in office workers. They need to sit for a long time due to work. This will cause the hip blood to run poorly, which leads to accumulation of a lot of fat in the waist, buttocks, thighs and other parts. If you have the habit of crossing your legs, it will affect the blood circulation of the legs, resulting in swelling of the lower body, and the problem of increasing fat thickness, which will form a pear-shaped body. Compared with non-obese people, pear-shaped obesity still has a serious risk, only slightly smaller than apple-shaped obesity.

3.肥胖的危害

Dangers of Obesity

(1)肥胖者易出现代谢性疾病

Obese People Are Prone to Metabolic Diseases

肥胖者的糖尿病患病发生率显著高于常人。有研究显示，在Ⅱ型糖尿病中80%都是肥胖者，且发生肥胖时间越长，患有糖尿病的概率就越大。肥胖者，特别是苹果形肥胖者，由于进食脂肪多、体内脂肪储存多、高胰岛素血症可增高血脂、血脂的清除等原因，所以比普通人更容易表现为血脂紊乱。

The incidence of diabetes in obese people is significantly higher than that of ordinary people. Studies have shown that 80 percent of people with type 2 diabetes are obese, and the longer the obesity occurs, the greater the chance of suffering from diabetes. Obese people, especially those with apple-shaped obesity, are more prone to dyslipidemia than ordinary people. They are more likely to show dyslipidemia than ordinary people because of taking in more fat, storing more fat in the body, hyperinsulinemia and clear of blood lipids.

(2)肥胖者易出现皮肤病

Obese People Are Prone to Skin Diseases

肥胖者常患对磨疹，多发于头部、腋窝等皮肤皱褶处，造成红色发痒的湿疹，且常在腰部、大腿等处出现妊娠纹样的线纹，称为肥胖纹，是由于真皮组织迅速生长时断裂所产生。另外，由于心脏肥大，静脉血液回流慢，亦容易导致静脉曲张。

Obese people often suffer from abrasion, which occurs in the skin folds of the head and armpits. It causes red and itchy eczema, and pregnancy-like lines that often appear on the waist, thighs, etc. Pregnancy-like lines are also called obesity lines, which is caused by the breakage of the dermal tissue during rapid growth.

In addition, due to cardiac hypertrophy, venous blood return is slowed, which can easily lead to varicose veins.

（3）肥胖与高血压密切相关

Obesity Is Closely Related to Hypertension

肥胖者容易患高血压，有的肥胖人群会出现血压波动；20~30岁的肥胖者，高血压的发生率要比同年龄而正常体重者高1倍；40~50岁的肥胖者，高血压的发生概率要比非肥胖者高50%。一个中度肥胖（BMI>30）的人，发生高血压的概率是体重正常者的5倍多。

Obese people are prone to hypertension, and some obese people will have blood pressure fluctuations. Obese people between 20 and 30 years old have twice the incidence of hypertension than those of the same age and normal weight. Obese people between 40 and 50 years old have a higher incidence of hypertension, which is 50% higher than that of non-obese people. A person with moderate obesity (BMI>30) is more than 5 times more likely to develop high blood pressure than a person with normal weight.

（4）肥胖易增加心脑血管疾病的风险

Obesity Easily Increases the Risk of Heart and Cerebrovascular Diseases

首先，肥胖人群容易发生大动脉粥样硬化，他们的脑血管又硬又脆，容易在高血压的作用下发生破裂，引起脑出血，甚至危及生命。其次，肥胖者血液中的异常因子也比普通人高，这种因子使血栓一旦生成就难以溶解，所以肥胖者容易发生脑梗死。而过多的脂质沉积在动脉壁内，致使管腔狭窄、硬化，易发生冠心病、心绞痛，同时由于肥胖者增加心脏血液流通负担导致心功能衰竭。

First of all, obese people are prone to large atherosclerosis. Their cerebral blood vessels are hard and fragile, and they are prone to rupture under the action of high blood pressure, causing cerebral hemorrhage and even threatening people's life. Secondly, the abnormal factor in the blood of obese people is also higher than that of ordinary people. This factor makes it difficult to dissolve thrombus once it is formed, so obese people are prone to cerebral infarction. Excessive lipid deposits in the wall of arteries cause stenosis and hardening of the lumen, which make people become prone to coronary heart disease and angina pectoris. At the same time, obese people increase the burden of heart blood flow and lead to heart failure.

（5）肥胖对后代健康有影响

Obesity Has Impact on the Health of Offspring

肥胖母亲的胎儿容易早产、先天畸形、巨大、围产期死亡等，也会增加孩子儿童期肥胖的概率。同时肥胖使得生育风险增加。

The fetus of obese mothers is prone to premature birth, congenital malformations, large size, and perinatal death. Mothers'obesity will also increase the chance of children's obesity in their childhood. At the same time, obesity increases the risk during the fertility.

（6）肥胖导致呼吸功能低下（气喘）

Obesity Leads to Respiratory Hypofunction (Asthma)

肥胖造成胸腹脂肪增厚，使肺容量下降、肺活量减少而影响肺部正常换气的功能。且因为换气不足，可能会造成血管堵塞。严重者可能发生肺性高血压、心脏梗死性心衰竭。因为脂肪的堆积，亦可能影响肺部气管内纤毛的活动，使其无法发挥正常功能。

Obesity causes thickening of chest and abdominal fat, which reduces lung capacity and lung capacity and affects the function of normal ventilation in the lungs. And because of insufficient ventilation, it may cause blockages in blood vessels. In severe cases, pulmonary hypertension and infarct heart failure may occur. Because of the accumulation of fat, it may also affect the movement of cilia in the lung trachea, making it unable to perform normal functions.

（7）胆结石、痛风、脂肪肝

Gallstones, Gout and Fatty Liver

有时食用过量有时饥饿并伴有肥胖现象，是胆石症与痛风的共同点。肥胖者与正常人相比，胆固醇含量增多，超过了胆汁中的溶解度，因此肥胖者容易并发高比例的胆固醇结石。

Sometimes eating more, sometimes keeping hunger, accompanied by obesity phenomenon, is the common ground of gallstone disease and gout. Compared with normal people, obese people have more cholesterol than the solubility in bile. Therefore, obese people are prone to a high proportion of cholesterol stones.

（8）肥胖易诱发癌症

Obesity Easily Induces Cancer

据英国著名医学杂志《柳叶刀》发表的大型流行病调查显示，在英国524万人群中发现，有17种癌症患病风险与肥胖明显相关，包括胆囊癌、甲状腺癌、肝癌、结肠癌、卵巢癌、乳腺癌等。

另外，肥胖可能引发一些社会和心理问题。近年肥胖人口的激增，不仅招致医疗费用负担增加，还增大了交通工具的燃料费支出，并使得二氧化碳排放增多。在心理上，肥胖人群普遍有较低的自尊，较高的焦虑与抑郁感。且人们通常对肥胖人群具有刻板印象，他们在工作面试上受到歧视；校园暴力对象的四之一是肥胖青少年；在约会市场上女性肥胖人群会受到更多打击等诸如此类。

According to a large-scale epidemiological survey published by the famous British medical journal The Lancet, among 5.24 million people in the UK, it was found that there are 17 types of cancer risk were significantly associated with obesity, including gallbladder cancer, thyroid cancer, liver cancer, colon cancer, ovarian cancer, breast cancer, etc.

What's more, fat may trigger some psychology and social problems. The recent surge in obesity has not only increased the burden of health care costs, but has also increased fuel costs for transportation and increased carbon dioxide emissions. Generally speaking, obese people have psychologically lower self-esteem and higher levels of anxiety and depression. And people often stereotype obese ones who are discriminated against in job interviews. Also, one in four of the targets of violence on campus is obese teens What's worse, women who are obese in the dating market are more likely to be dampened their enthusiasm, and so on.

4.导致肥胖的因素

Factors Leading to Obesity

（1）基因因素

Genetic Factor

科学家普遍将导致肥胖的基因因素定义为"多因素继承"。例如，非胰岛素依赖型糖尿病和肥胖都属于这种遗传。根据研究，父母中如果有一人是肥胖的，那他们的孩子会有40%的概率患上肥胖症。双亲若都是肥胖的，那么孩子肥胖的概率会上升至70%到80%。

Scientists generally define the genetic factors that contribute to obesity as "multifactorial inheritance". For example, both non-insulin-dependent diabetes and obesity belong to this kind of inheritance. According to the research, if one of the parents is obese, the child has a 40% chance of obesity. If both parents are obese, the chance will increase to 70%–80%.

（2）饮食因素

Dietary Factor

在当今社会，丰富多样的食物已成了导致肥胖的主要因素。热量摄入过多，尤其是高脂肪饮食是造成肥胖病的主要原因。脂肪进入血液后，一部分供给身体活动所需要的热量，一部分作为细胞的组成部分，还有一部分转化为其他物质，多余的便进入脂肪库储存起来。如果吃得太多，机体所摄取的热量超过正常的消耗，食物中的脂肪进入脂肪库储存的数量就会增多，从而形成肥胖。

In today's society, abundant and diverse foods have become the main factors leading to obesity. Excessive calorie intake, especially high-fat diet, is the main cause of obesity. After fat enters the human blood, a part of it provides the calories needed for physical activity, a part of it is used as a component of cells, and the rest is converted into other substance. Then the surplus will enter the fat bank and be stored. If you eat too much and the body's intake of calories exceeds normal consumption, the amount of fat in the food stored in the human fat depot will increase, resulting in obesity.

（3）心理因素

Psychological Factor

控制饮食的中枢的功能通常受制于精神状态，当神经兴奋而激素分泌增多时，易致肥胖。精神高度紧张，交感神经兴奋时，食欲被抑制。很多人为了解除心情上的烦恼、情绪上的不稳定，用"吃"来作为发泄，这也能导致体重超标。

The center that controls diet is usually restricted by the mental state. When the nerve is excited and the hormone increases, it's easy to lead to obesity. When the spirit is in high tension and sympathetic nervous excitement, appetite will be suppressed. Many people eat to vent their anxieties and emotional instability, which can lead to their overweight.

（4）生活习惯因素

Living Habits Factors

随着交通工具发达、工作机械化、家务量减轻等，使得人体消耗热量的机会减少。因此，人们变得慵懒，日常活动趋于缓慢，再次减低热量的消耗，导致恶性循环，助长肥胖的发生。缺乏睡眠也是可能导致肥胖的因素之一。研究发现，如果缺眠的话，人体的整体胰岛素反应能力就会下降16%，胃部脂肪细胞对胰岛素的灵敏性下降了30%，这一水平通常只会出现在患肥胖症和糖尿病病人身上。所以长期睡眠不足，也就会发胖，甚至患上糖尿病。

With the development of transportation, the mechanization of work, and the reduction of household chores, the human body has less chance of consuming heat. Accordingly, people become lazy. Their daily activities tend to slow, thus reducing the consumption of heat again, which brings about a vicious circle to abet the occurrence of obesity. Lack of sleep is also one of the factors that may lead to obesity. Studies have found that if sleep is absent, the body's overall insulin response capacity will drop by 16%, and the sensitivity of stomach fat cells to insulin will drop by 30%. This level usually only appears in patients with obesity and diabetes. Therefore, if you lack sleep for a long time, you will get fat and even suffer from diabetes.

（三）科学减肥，达到健康

1.控制体重的本质

Essence of Weight Control

控制体重的本质在于保持能量代谢的平衡，即平衡能量摄入和消耗。抑制肥胖有一个原则，就是让能量代谢处于负平衡状态。

Remember that the essence of weight control is to maintain the balance of energy metabolism, that is, to balance energy intake and expenditure. The principle of obesity control is the negative balance of energy metabolism.

2. 科学减肥，达到健康的方法

Scientific Method to Lose Weight and Achieve Health

科学减肥，达到健康的方法在于合理饮食和定期运动。

So how to scientifically lose weight and achieve health? The answer is proper eating and regular exercise.

（1）科学饮食

Scientific Diet

科学的饮食是达到健康的重要途径。对于担心药物减肥的副作用者，最好的减肥原则就是通过饮食控制达到减肥目的。合理选择食物主要从以下三个方面入手，即均衡饮食、控制总热量以及规律饮食。遵循以下几点饮食原则，不仅能全面均衡地摄入营养，同时也有利于科学减肥，达到健康。

Scientific diet is one of the most important way to achieve health. For those who are worried about the side effects of the drug weight loss, the best weight loss principle is to achieve weight loss through diet control. By following the following dietary principles, we can not only absorb nutrition in a comprehensive and balanced way, but also help to lose weight scientifically and achieve health.

①均衡饮食

Balanced Diet

膳食均衡是营养科学的一个重要长远的目标。除了出生至六个月之内的婴儿用母乳喂养可以获取均衡的膳食以外，可以说没有单一的食物能称得上是人类的均衡膳食，只有相互搭配的多种食物才可以构成实际生活中的均衡的膳食。膳食必须符合个体生长发育和生理状况等特点，含有人体所需要的各种营养成分，含量适当，全面满足身体需要，维持正常生理功能，促进生长发育和健康，这种膳食称为"均衡膳食"。

A balanced diet is an important long-term goal of nutritional science. There is no single food that can be called a balanced human diet, except for a well-balanced diet for babies who are breast-fed between birth and six months of age. Only a variety of foods can constitute the actual life and you must mix them reasonably. A balanced diet must conform to the characteristics of individual growth and development and physiological conditions, contain various nutrients required by the human body, which have appropriate content. It could fully meet the needs of the body, maintain normal physiological functions as well as promote personal growth, development and health. This diet is what we call a "balanced diet".

②体重控制的膳食规定

Rules for Weight Control

许多人认为营养过剩会导致肥胖。然而，真正导致肥胖的是额外的热量摄入。以下是体重控制的膳食规定：

Many people believe that overnutrition can lead to obesity. However, what really causes obesity is the extra calorie intake. The following are dietary rules for weight control:

首先，应该限制饮食热量，以达到负能量的平衡。每天减少500~700卡路里的能量摄入，这样可以在10~14天内减少1千克脂肪。其次，我们要妥善分配摄入的营养。提高蛋白质的质量，并为身体补充微量元素。三餐热能比应当控制在4：4：2。再者，注意多饮水，因为缺水会加快体内脂肪的积累。最后，持续的饮食控制是至关重要的因素。

First, we should limit dietary calories to reach the balance of negative energy. Reducing energy intake by five hundred to seven hundred calories per day can reduce one kilogram of fat in ten to fourteen days. Second, we should get an appropriate nutrition distribution, including improving protein in quality and supplying trace elements to your body as well. The ratio of the calory between three meals need to be controlled at four to four than two (4:4:2). And again, don't forget to drink enough water: because lack of water will promote fat accumulation in the body. Finally, consistent diet control is the most critical factor.

（2）定期运动

Regular Exercise

俗话说，保持运动健康在，不让病魔闯进来。因为运动可以提升肌肉燃烧脂肪的能力，提高身体利用脂肪能量的比例，增加基础消耗量，这些都是减肥所必需的。一般运动分为两种，一种是有氧运动，另一种是无氧运动。选择不同种类的运动，其锻炼效果也不一样。

As the saying goes, keeping exercising can remain healthy and prevent illness. Because exercise can improve the ability of muscles to burn fat, increase the proportion of fat energy used by the body, and increase basic consumption, all of which are necessary for weight loss. There are two kinds of exercises, one is aerobic exercise and the other is anaerobic exercise. Choosing different types of exercise, and the exercise effect you'll get is also different.

①有氧运动

Aerobic exercise

有氧运动是指人体在氧气充分供应的情况下进行的运动。有氧运动的运动强度应保持在中等水平，这就意味着最适合运动的心率，即靶心率（目标心率），应为140次/分钟~160次/分钟。靶心率等于心率储备乘以60%~80%再加上安静心率。同时，心率储备可以用最大心率减去安静心率来得到；而最大心率又等于220减去我们的年龄。

Aerobic exercise refers to the movement of the body in the condition of sufficient oxygen supply. The exercise intensity of aerobic exercise should be maintained at a moderate level, which means that the most suitable heart rate for exercise, that is, the target heart rate (target heart rate), should be 140 to 160 beats per minute. The target heart rate is equal to the heart rate reserve multiplied by 60% to 80% plus the resting heart rate. At the same time, the heart rate reserve can be obtained by subtracting the resting heart rate from the maximum heart rate; and the maximum heart rate is equal to 220 minus our age.

例如：某人40岁，安静时的心率为80次/分钟。其最大心率为180，心率储备为100。所以，他最合适的运动心率是140次/分钟，即等于100乘以60%，然后加80次/分钟，之后160次/分钟，则是通过100乘以80%，然后加80次/分钟。所以，只要他能把心率控制在140次/分钟~160次/分钟，那么他就处于自己最好的运动状态。当然，如果运动强度过低，那么运动效果可能会减弱，而运动强度过大，身体的负担就会过重。

For example: someone is 40 years old and has a heart rate of 80 beats per minute at rest. Its maximum heart rate is 180, and its heart rate reserve is 100. Therefore, his most suitable exercise heart rate is 140 beatsperminute, which is equal to 100 times 60%, then add 80 beatsperminute, and then 160 beatsperminute, it is through 100 times 80%, and then add 80 timesperminute. So, as long as he manages to control his heart rate between 140 to 160 times, then he is in his own perfect condition for exercise. Of course, if the exercise intensity is too low, then the effect of exercise may be weakened while the exercise being too intensive, the burden on the body will be too heavy.

②无氧运动

Anaerobics

无氧运动是指人体肌肉在无氧供能代谢状态下进行的运动。它们大多是负荷强度大、瞬时性强的运动，难以长时间维持。

Anaerobics refers to exercise under the circumstance of insufficient oxygen metabolism. Most of them are exercise with high load intensity and strong instantaneity, so it is difficult to do those kinds of exercise for a long time.

③运动处方

Exercise Prescription

以下是一个简单的运动处方，它可以帮助你通过锻炼来控制体重。该处方由两部分组成，即有氧运动和无氧运动。该处方更适合健康的中青年，对于老年人和体弱者应慎用。

Here is a simple exercise prescription, which can help you control your weight through exercise. The prescription consists of two parts, including aerobic exercise and anaerobic exercise. The prescription is more suitable for healthy young and middle-aged. It should be used with caution in the elderly and the infirm.

适量的抗阻力量训练和伸展练习能提高基础代谢率；而大强度间歇性训练HIIT（High Intensity Intermittent Training）则有利于大量动员脂肪。最有效的体重控制方法是有氧运动和无氧运动相结合。无氧运动先于有氧运动，前者消耗糖原，而后者消耗更多的脂肪。

Moderate resistance training and stretching exercise can improve the basic metabolic rate, while High Intensity Intermittent Training (HIIT) could be conducive to the mobilization of large amounts of fat. So the most effective method of weight control is the combination of aerobics and anaerobics. Anaerobics goes before aerobics, as the former consume glycogen and the latter consume more fat.

比如，在准备花一小时进行运动的情况下，先做10分钟的无氧运动以基础糖原，再花50分钟进行有氧运动，比单纯地花一小时进行有氧运动的效果更好。

For example, if you're going to spend an hour exercising, do anaerobics of 10 minutes first, which can consume your basic glycogen and then do aerobics in 50 minutes, it will be better compared with you simply spending an hour doing aerobics.

在执行运动处方前，应当选择好可以安排锻炼的时间，最好是在午饭前。在锻炼过程中应当循序渐进。

Before administering an exercise prescription, you should choose a time when you can do exercise, preferably before lunch. The exercise process should be gradual.

④关于运动减肥的误区

Misunderstandings about Weight Loss

有些人认为不透气的服装，比如桑拿服，有益减肥。但事实上，出汗并不一定意味着减肥；还有观点认为出汗越多，效果越好，这也是不对的。运动强度需要根据个人身体情况而定，超过一定的运动强度反而会适得其反。而有些人认为锻炼30分钟以下就好，其实对于有氧运动来说，一般30分钟有氧才起效，前面燃烧的都是糖原，30分钟后才开始燃烧脂肪，运动时间必须达到30分钟以上，60分钟左右为宜。当然，锻炼者的首要任务应当是找到最适合自身的运动方式，而不是相信只有特定的运动才能帮助减肥。尽量选择喜欢并能长时间坚持的运动，运动频率可以根据具体目标而定，一般一周3~5次为宜。

Some people think that wearing impermeable clothes like sauna clothes are good for it. But in fact, sweating does not necessarily mean losing fat. The idea that the more you sweat, the better, is also not true. The intensity of exercise needs to be based on the individual's physical condition, and exceeding a certain intensity of exercise can be counterproductive. And some people just work out less than 30 mins, which is not useful for fat to burn after 30 min cardio. Glucagon is the only thing got consumed in the first half of hour. Therefore, exercise time in more than 30 minutes and 60 minutes is much more appropriate. Of course, your priority should be finding the way of exercise that suits you most instead of believing that only a certain kind of exercise can help you to lose weight. Try to choose the exercise that you like and can persist for a long time. The frequency of exercise can be determined according to the specific goal. And we recommend the frequency of exercise is 3 to 5 times a week.

第二节 营养与体能
Section Two Nutrition and Physical Agility

一、七大营养素
Seven Nutrients

研究表明，人类为了维持正常的生命活动，必须不断从外界摄入必要的物质，用以供给能量、构成机体组织、调节生理活动等。这些所摄取的必要物质被称为营养素，主要包含水、蛋白质、脂肪、糖类、维生素、矿物质、纤维素七大类。七大营养素存在于各类食品中，每类营养素在人体内所起的作用不同，需要的含量也不同，任意一种营养素过多或不足都会影响人体正常的新陈代谢而损害健康。

Researches show that in order to maintain normal life activities, humans must constantly take in necessary substances from the outside world to supply energy, form body tissues, and regulate physiological activities. These necessary substances ingested are called nutrients, which mainly include seven categories of water, protein, fat, sugar, vitamins, minerals, and cellulose. The seven major nutrients exist in various foods. Each type of nutrient plays a different role in the human body and requires a different content. Too much or insufficient of any one nutrient will affect the normal metabolism of the human body and damage health.

二、体能

Fitness

体能也叫体适能，主要通过体育锻炼而获得。保持良好的体能可以使我们的身体更健康，寿命能延长，生命更有价值。每个人要获得健康都需要有一定的体能，良好的体能与长期锻炼、科学的饮食方法、良好的口腔卫生、足够时间的休息和放松等都有密切的关系。

Fitness is also called physical fitness, which is mainly obtained through exercise. Keeping good fitness can make our body healthier, life span longer and life more valuable. Everyone needs a certain fitness to get healthy. Good fitness is related closely to long-term exercise, scientific diet, good oral health, enough time to rest and relax.

（一）分类

Classification

体能可以分为两类：与健康有关的体能和与运动技能有关的体能。

There are two type of fitness which are health-related and motor-skill-related.

1. 与健康有关的体能

Health-related Fitness

（1）心肺耐力

Cardiopulmonary Endurance

心肺耐力指一个人持续身体活动的能力。心肺和血管的功能对于氧和营养物的分配、清除体内垃圾具有重要的作用。心肺功能越强，走、跑、学习和工作就会越轻松，进行各种活动保持的时间也会越长。

The first is cardiopulmonary endurance, which refers to a person's ability to keep physical activity. Cardiopulmonary and vascular functions play an important role in the distribution of oxygen and nutrients, and in the removal of waste. The stronger the cardiopulmonary function, the easier it will be to walk, run, study and work, and the longer it will take to maintain various activities.

（2）柔韧性

Body Flexibility

柔韧性是指身体各个关节的活动幅度以及跨过关节的肌肉、肌腱、韧带、皮肤和其他组织的弹性和伸展能力，我们可以通过经常性的身体练习进而提高。柔韧性是绝大多数的锻炼项目所必需的体能成分之一，对于提高身体活动水平、预防肌肉紧张以及保持良好的体态等具有重要作用。

Body flexibility refers to the range of movement of each joint of the body, as well as the elasticity and stretching ability of muscles, tendons, ligaments, skin and other tissues across the joint. We can improve it through regular exercises. Body flexibility is one of the necessary physical components in most exercise programs, which plays an important role in improving the level of physical activity, preventing muscle tension and maintaining good body type.

（3）肌肉力量

Muscular Strength

肌肉力量，顾名思义，是肌肉群一次竭尽全力从事抵抗阻力的活动能力。所有的身体活动均需要使用力量，哪怕是站立或走路。肌肉强壮有助于预防关节的扭伤、肌肉的疼痛和身体的疲劳。需注意的是，我们不能只强调某一肌肉群发展，而忽视另一肌肉群的发展，这样会影响身体的结构和我们的形态。

The third is muscular strength, the ability of muscle groups to make maximal effort to resist external resistance forces. Strength is required for all the physical activity, even standing or walking. Strong muscle helps prevent joint sprains, muscle pain, and body fatigue. It should be noted that we can not only emphasize the development of one muscle group, but ignore another, which will affect the structure of the body and our shape.

(4) 肌肉耐力

Muscular Endurance

肌肉耐力指一块肌肉或肌肉群在一段时间内重复进行肌肉收缩的能力，它与肌肉力量密切相关。一个肌肉强壮并且耐力好的人更易抵御疲劳的发生，因为这样的人只需要花很少的力气就可以重复收缩肌肉。

The fourth is muscular endurance, which refers to the ability of a muscle or muscle group to repeatedly perform muscle contraction in a period. It is closely related to muscular strength. A person with strong muscles and good endurance is more likely to resist fatigue, because such a person can repeatedly contract muscles with little effort.

(5) 身体成分

Body Composition

身体成分包括肌肉、骨骼、脂肪和其他等。其中，体能与体内脂肪比例之间的关系最为密切，脂肪过多者是不健康的，其在活动时比其他人需要消耗更多的能量，心肺功能的负担也更重，所以，我们心脏病和高血压发生的可能性更大。另外，肥胖也会使人的心理健康水平下降，寿命也会因此缩短。要维持适宜的体内脂肪，就必须注意能量吸收和能量消耗之间的平衡，而通过体育锻炼也可以控制脂肪增加，所谓"管住嘴，迈开腿"就是这个道理。

The last category is body composition, including muscle, bone, fat and others. Among them, the relationship between fitness and the proportion of fat in the body is the closest. People with too much fat are not healthy. They need to consume more energy than other people when they exercise, and the burden of cardiopulmonary function is heavier. Therefore, we are more likely to have heart disease and high blood pressure. In addition, obesity will also reduce people's mental health and life expectancy. In order to maintain the proper body fat, we must pay attention to the balance between energy absorption and consumption, and we can also control the increase of fat through exercise. The so-called saying "exercise more and eat less" is the truth.

2.与动作技能有关的体能

Motor-skill-related Fitness

（1）速度

Speed

速度指快速完成某项运动的能力。常表现为反应快慢。单个动作完成的时间、重复动作的频率以及整体移动的速度等。但是，它们都依赖于反应的速度和肌肉收缩的速度之和。

Speed refers to the ability to complete an exercise quickly. It is often manifested as fast or slow response. The time to complete a single action, the frequency of repeated actions, and the speed of the overall movement. However, they all depend on the sum of the speed of reaction and the speed of muscle contraction.

（2）力量

Strength

力量是指用肌肉单位或肌肉单位的组合施加力的能力，可以通过能完成的动作的难度来测定。各项运动都极重视力量的训练，提高力量素质就是要发育肌肉并提高神经调节机能。

Strength refers to the ability to exert force with muscle units or a combination of muscle units, and can be measured by difficulty of the completed movement. All sports attach great importance to strength training. To improve strength quality is to develop muscles and neuroregulation.

（3）灵敏性

Agility

灵敏性指在活动过程中，既快速又准确地变化身体移动方向的能力。一个人是否灵敏，很大程度上依赖于神经肌肉的协调性和反应时间，所以可以通过提高这两方面的能力来改善人体的灵敏性。

The third is agility, which refers to the ability to change the direction of body movement quickly and accurately in the process of activity. Whether a person is agility or not depends on the coordination and reaction time of neuromuscular to a great extent, so we can improve the sensitivity by improving these two abilities.

（4）神经肌肉协调性
Neuromuscular Coordination

神经肌肉协调性，主要反映一个人的视觉、听觉和平衡觉与熟练的动作技能相结合的能力。在球类运动中，需要近乎同时看球、判断方向、完成动作，使得这种体能成分显得尤为重要。

The fourth is neuromuscular coordination, which primarily reflects a person's ability to combine vision, hearing, and balance with skilled motor skills. In ball games, it is necessary to watch the ball, judge the direction and complete the action at the same time, which makes this physical component particularly important.

（5）平衡
Balance

平衡指当运动或静止站立时保持身体稳定性的能力。滑冰、滑雪、体操、舞蹈等项目对于提高平衡能力是很好的运动，闭目单足站立练习也有相当好的效果。

The fifth is balance, which refers to the ability to maintain body stability when moving or standing. Skating, skiing, gymnastics, dance and other events are good sports for improving the balance ability, and standing on one leg with eyes closed also has a good effect.

（6）反应时
Reaction Time

反应时指对某些外部刺激做出生理反应的时间。反应快速是许多项目优秀运动员的特征，特别是在短跑的起跑阶段，反应时的作用更大。

Finally, reaction time refers to the time of physiological response to some external stimulus. Quick reaction is the characteristic of many excellent athletes. It plays a more important role especially in the launching phase of sprint.

三、营养与体能的关系
The Relationship between Nutrition and Physical Fitness

糖和脂肪是供能的主要物质。例如，在高强度、短时间的运动（如速度、力量项目）中，主要由糖供能，在长时间、低强度的运动（如耐力项目）中，主要由脂肪提供能量。

Carbohydrates and fats are the main substances for energy. For example, in high-intensity and short-term exercises (such as speed and strength events), energy is mainly provided by carbohydrates! By contrast in long-term and low-intensity exercises (such as endurance events), energy is mainly provided by fat.

（一）糖与体能的关系

Relationship between Carbohydrates and Physical Fitness

运动中能量消耗的增加，会加大对能量的需求。体育锻炼中提供人体能量的主要物质是糖和脂肪，在高强度和长时间的运动中，肝脏和肌肉中糖可降低到临界水平。糖作为能源在运动中起到关键的作用，运动强度决定了糖和脂肪哪个是运动中的主要能量来源。所以我们可以增加膳食中多糖的比例，并控制脂肪摄入，就能够保证肌肉和肝脏中糖的供能，来满足大强度运动的需要。

The increase in energy consumption during exercise will increase the demand for energy. The main substances that provide human energy in physical exercise are carbohydrates and fat. During high-intensity and long-term exercise, the carbohydrates in the liver and muscle can be reduced to a critical level. Carbohydrates plays a key role in exercise as an energy source. Exercise intensity determines whether sugar or fat is the main source of energy during exercise. Therefore, we can increase the proportion of polysaccharides in the diet and control the fat intake to ensure the supply of carbohydrates in the muscles and liver to meet the needs of high-intensity exercise.

（二）蛋白质与体能的关系

Relationship between Protein and Physical Fitness

蛋白质的基本功能是组成和修补人体组织，但当糖不足或应激状态时，它也能作为能源物质提供能量。从事力量训练者需要合理膳食宝塔中的各种食物，而不是简单的额外补充蛋白质。在进行力量训练的人不仅要补充三大营养素，也要补充促进能量产生所需要的微量营养素。

The basic function of protein is to form and repair human tissues, but when carbohydrates is insufficient or under stress, it can also provide energy as well. Those engaged in strength training need to eat a variety of foods in the pagoda, rather than simply taking extra protein. People who are doing strength training must not only supplement the three major nutrients, but also get the micronutrients needed to promote energy production.

（三）维生素与体能的关系

Relationship between Vitamins and Physical Fitness

维生素与体能也有密不可分的关系。我们一般认为，运动增加了能量需要，而维生素具有分解食物转化为能量的作用，所以额外补充维生素能够促进能量的产生。但其实，大剂量地补充维生素可能造成维生素和其他微量营养素之间的平衡的失调，甚至导致维生素的中毒反应的出现，所以补充维生素要注意适量。

Vitamins are also closely related to physical fitness. We generally believe that exercise increases energy requirements, and vitamins can break down food into energy, so additional vitamin supplements can promote energy production. But in fact, supplementing vitamins in large doses may cause an imbalance between vitamins and other micronutrients, and even lead to the emergence of vitamin poisoning reactions, so you should pay attention to appropriate amounts of vitamin supplements.

（四）抗氧化剂与体能的关系

Relationship between Antioxidant and Physical Fitness

近年来有研究发现，某些维生素和一些无机盐有新的功能，这些无机盐和维生素可作为抗氧化剂对细胞具有保护作用。抗氧化剂其实是一种可以阻止氧对细胞损害的化学物质，即阻止氧自由基对细胞的攻击。

In recent years, studies have found that certain vitamins and some inorganic salts have new functions. These inorganic salts and vitamins can act as antioxidants to protect cells. Antioxidant is actually a chemical substance that can prevent oxygen from damaging cells, that is, prevent oxygen free radicals from attacking cells.

思考

Questions

1. 如何预防和控制成人肥胖症？

How to prevent and control adult obesity?

2. 为什么有时没吃早饭去上课会觉得头晕眼花、四肢无力？

Why do I sometimes feel dizzy and weak when I go to class without breakfast?

3. 请按照有氧无氧运动相结合的特征，给自己制定一份减肥最佳的运动处方。

Please design an optimal exercise prescription for weight loss based on characteristics of the combination of aerobic and anaerobic exercise.

第三章　体育锻炼与心理、社会健康
CHAPTER THREE EXERCISE AND MENTAL & SOCIAL HEALTH

随着现代社会的发展，生活节奏加快，竞争日趋激烈，心理健康和社会健康逐渐成为人们关注的焦点问题。体育活动既是身心活动也是社会活动，进行体育锻炼不仅有利于身心健康，而且对人的社会健康具有积极的促进作用。本章对体育锻炼、心理健康、社会健康、应激做了系统性概述，并对体育锻炼如何影响心理健康、社会健康、应激做了详细介绍。学习本章内容，有助于培养良好的健康意识，形成终身锻炼的习惯。

With the development of modern society, the pace of life is accelerating, and the social competition is becoming increasingly fierce. Mental health and social health have gradually become the focus of people's attention. Physical exercise is a physical and mental activity and a social activity which is not only beneficial to physical and mental health, but also has a positive role in promoting one's social health. This chapter gives a systematic overview on physical exercise, mental health, social health and stress. Detailed introduction of how physical exercise affects mental health, social health and stress will be demonstrated. Through the study of this chapter, good health awareness can be cultivated and the habit of lifelong exercise can be formed.

第一节 体育锻炼与心理健康
Section One Exercise and Mental Health

一、体育锻炼
Exercise

（一）体育锻炼的定义
Definition of Exercise

卡斯帕森等（1985）指出体育锻炼/体育运动是身体活动的一部分，具有计划性、结构化和重复性，并且以改善或维持身体素质为最终或中间的目标，而身体素质则是一组与健康或技能相关的属性。联合国教科文组织颁布的《体育运动国际宪章》（1978）中，对体育与体育运动做了界定。其认为体育是一种人权，是提高生活质量的手段，体育运动是教育与文化的一个基本方面。就此概念，杨文轩（1996）指出，体育运动有助于个人维持和增进健康，使人克服现代生活所带来的弊端，带给人一种有益的享受。同时，体育运动也可以丰富社会交往活动并培养人们公平公正的体育精神。

Caspersen et al. (1985) pointed out that exercise is a planned, structured, and repeated physical activity with the aim to improve or maintain physical fitness. In the definition of the International Charter of Physical Education, Physical Activity and Sport promulgated by UNESCO in 1978, the practice of physical education and exercise is a fundamental right for all, as a means of promoting life quality and a basic element of education and culture.

Based on this concept, Yang Wenxuan (1996) pointed out that exercise can help individuals maintain and improve their health, help people overcome the disadvantages in modern life, and offer people beneficial enjoyment. At the same time, exercise can also enrich social activities and cultivate people's fair sportsmanship.

（二）体育锻炼与徒步步数
Exercise and Walking Steps

日常生活中最简单的锻炼方式就是步行。随着微信在我国普及，微信运动也有了越来越多的用户。自从微信推出了可以记录每日步数的功能，朋友圈就掀起了一阵晒步数的风潮，一时间所有人都变成了运动达人。

The simplest form of exercise in daily life is walking. As WeChat is popularized in our country, there is an increased number of people beginning to use Wechat Motion. Since WeChat published such a function to record daily steps, the Moments section in WeChat has witnessed an upsurge of demonstrating one's daily steps, as if everybody becomes exercise lovers overnight.

不管男女老少都先后开始暴走，每天都在为了登顶步数排行榜增加运动量，积攒步数。1万步是最低的，2万步才能进入排行榜的前几名，甚至大晚上也要出去溜达一圈，直到自己的头像再次霸占微信运动封面才停止。这场盛大的全民暴走热潮，也让越来越多的人开始重视自己的日常运动量。

Regardless of gender and age, everyone is scrambling to walk. They increase their amount of exercise and accumulate steps to rank first in the Moments. From then on, ten thousand steps a day is just a basic requirement if you want your name on the board, and only by making at least 20000 steps will you have your chance to be ranked first. Even late at night, people will also go out and walk to ensure his or her crowning of Wechat Motion. This grand national upsurge also let more and more people begin to pay more attention on their daily exercise.

美国卫生与公众服务部（2001）也明确指出，成年人每天应至少步行1万步。有人可能会认为走1万步并不困难，去厨房接水，到街对面吃饭，这些日常行为都是增加步数的简易方法。但是，有一个概念需要大家明确：日常生活中的步数并不等于锻炼的步数，生活步数是指我们日常生活中无法避免的步行运动。比如下楼取快递，下班后吃饭购物等。这些步行运动由于速度慢、强度低、没有连续性、姿态不正确，而不能算是真正的运动。只有日常集中时间来进行步行锻炼，并且保持中速走（90~120步/分）才是最有效的步行健身运动。（美国运动医学会推荐）

US Department of Health and Human Services (2001) also clearly pointed out that an adult should walk at least 10000 steps per day. Some people may argue that walking 10000 steps is not difficult. Pouring a cup of water in kitchen, having lunch across the street... All of these can easily add up to a lot of walking. Howerer, it should be pointed out that the number of steps in our daily life does not equal the number of steps in exercise. The number of steps in daily life refers to the inevitable walking activities in our daily life, such as fetching your package downstairs, picking up your takeout, and eating and shopping after work, etc. These walking activities cannot be considered as a way of exercise due to their low speed, low intensity, lack of continuity and incorrect walking posture. Only through a continuous time with the proper speed of 90 to 120 steps per minute can walking become the most effective form of exercise (recommended by the American College of Sports Medicine).

（三）体育锻炼的益处

Benefits of Exercise

人体由神经系统、循环系统、呼吸系统、运动系统、消化系统、排泄系统、生殖系统、内分泌和感觉器官组成。体育锻炼是由人体各器官系统协调配合所完成，同时，体育锻炼又对各器官系统产生良好影响。

The human body is composed of nervous system, circulatory system, respiratory system, motor system, digestive system, excretory system, reproductive system, endocrine system and sensory organs. Exercise is completed by the coordination and cooperation of the organ system of the human body. At the same time, exercise has a good effect on the organ system.

1. 改善运动系统功能

Improvement on Motor System

人体长期坚持体育锻炼，能增强骨组织的新陈代谢，改善骨的血液供应，可使骨密度增厚，提高骨关节的灵活性和柔韧性，可使肌纤维增粗，肌肉毛细血管增多，改善骨骼肌的供血功能，从而有效地提高和保持运动系统的能力。

Long-term exercise can enhance the metabolism of bone tissue, improve the blood supply of bone, increase bone density, enhance the flexibility and suppleness of bone joints, thicken muscle fibers, increase muscle capillaries, improve the blood supply function of skeletal muscle, and thus effectively improve and maintain the motor system function.

2. 改善心血管系统功能

Improvement on the Cardiovascular System

体育锻炼可以改善血管壁和血管的分布，心脏的容积增大，冠脉循环血量增加，提高脉搏输出量，增强身体活动能力，改善血压，减少心血管疾病，有效地降低糖尿病的发病风险。

Exercise can improve the distribution of blood vessel walls and the distribution of vessels, increase the heart volume and the blood volume of coronary circulation, improve cardial output, enhance physical mobility, improve blood pressure and reduce the risks of cardiovascular disease. It can also effectively reduce the risk of diabetes.

3. 改善呼吸系统功能

Improvement on Respiratory System

体育锻炼可以增加运动时的吸氧量，增强呼吸肌力量，提高肺泡的换气效率，增大肺活量，提高呼吸机能。

Exercise can increase the amount of oxygen inhaled during exercise, enhance respiratory muscle strength, improve the air exchange efficiency of alveolar ventilation, increase vital capacity, and improve respiratory function.

4. 改善消化系统功能

Improvement on Digestive System

体育锻炼可以促使消化腺分泌消化液，增强消化道的蠕动，改善胃肠的血液循环，提高肝脏机能，使食物的消化和营养物质的吸收更加顺利和充分。

Exercise can promote the secretion of digestive fluid, enhance the efficiency of the digestive tract, improve the blood circulation of the stomach and intestines, and the function of the liver, leading to better food digestion and nutrition absorption.

5. 改善神经系统和内分泌系统功能
Improvement on Nervous and Endocrine System

体育锻炼可以提高神经系统的灵活性、协调性和准确性，提高分析综合能力，缓解人体紧张情绪，提高生命活力，改善大脑和中枢神经系统的能量与氧气供应，促进思维和智力的发展，同时对人体的各种腺体结构和机能产生良好的影响。

Exercise can improve the flexibility, coordination and accuracy of the nervous system, improve comprehensive analysis ability, alleviate tension, improve life vitality, improve the energy and oxygen supply for brain and central nervous system and oxygen supply, and promote the development of thinking and intelligence, as well as lead to beneficial influence on body glands.

6. 改善免疫系统的功能
Improvement on Immune System

适量运动能提高免疫球蛋白水平，增加血液中白细胞的数量，增强呼吸道抗感染能力，预防和阻止病原菌的传播，运动产生的致热源可以抵抗外来病原体，抑制肿瘤细胞。

Moderate exercise can improve the level of immunoglobulin, increase leukocytes in the blood, reduce risks of infection on the respiratory tract, and prevent the spread of pathogenic bacteria. The heat generated through exercise can resist pathogens and inhibit tumor cells.

7. 提高人体适应能力
Improvement on Human Adaptability

人体适应能力包括人对外界自然环境的适应力，对疾病的抵抗力以及疾病损伤后的修复力。运动可以增强神经肌肉系统的协调能力，提高人体对外界刺激的适应能力和机体对致病因素的抵抗能力，全面提高人的体质水平。

Human adaptability includes the adaptability to the external natural environment, the resistance to disease and the ability to recover after the injury of disease. Exercise can enhance the coordination of the neuromuscular system, improve the adaptability to external stimuli and the resistance to pathogenic factors, and comprehensively promote physical fitness.

8. 改善人的精神状态和生活质量

Improvement on People's Mental Health and Life Quality

现代社会中频繁的人际交往和激烈的社会竞争，给人类造成了巨大的心理和精神压力。适当参加体育锻炼，可以调节人的神经和个人心理品质，转移人的注意力，改善人的精神和社会生活状态。

In modern society, frequent interpersonal communication and fierce social competition have caused great psychological pressure on human. Proper participation in exercise can regulate people's nerves and personal psychological status, divert people's attention, and improve people's mental health and social life.

（四）缺乏运动的影响

Effects of Lacking Exercise

据世界卫生组织统计，全球每年因缺乏运动而导致的死亡人数超过二百万。缺少锻炼会导致身体肥胖，体内寒气难以排出。例如在办公室久坐之后，会导致身体代谢速度减慢，皮肤松弛暗黄，没有弹性。此外，还会导致身体里的钙元素流失，从而手关节迟钝、骨质疏松、易出现疲劳感、毒素积压体内和便秘。也会出现一些口腔问题，例如口臭、牙龈肿痛等。

According to the World Health Organization, there are more than 2 million people die from lacking exercise. Lacking exercise can cause obesity and difficulties on draining cold type energy from your body. Sitting for a long time in the office will slow down metabolism, and the skin will become flabby and yellow without elasticity. One will also suffer from calcium loss, causing hand weakness, osteoporosis, fatigue, toxic overload and constipation. It can also cause oral illness, such as bad breath and gum disease, etc.

缺乏运动还会导致记忆衰退、抑郁症和失眠的概率提高，夜晚会出现疲劳却无法入睡的情况，从而逐渐损害身体器官的机能。心脏和肺功能也会受到不良影响，运动时易出汗和疲劳。消化系统特别是肠胃的功能也会变差，如食物消化吸收功能下降，食欲下降，拉肚子情况增加等。血液流通和心血管功能变差，导致四肢僵硬，出现头痛、头晕的症状。一些中老年人患上高血压、冠心病、痴呆症的概率也会提高，出现精神变差、黑眼圈加重的症状。抵抗力下降导致病毒入侵、体质变弱，做事没有精神的情况也会出现。儿童会生长缓慢，导致身材矮小。做运动时，也容易受伤，如韧带拉伤等。

Lacking exercise can also lead to a higher possibility of memory loss, depressionand insomnia. To Being in such condition for a long time, the function of organs can be damaged. With weakened cardiac function and pulmonary function, one can easily feel fatigue during exercise. The digestive system, especially the stomach and intestines, will deteriorate, causing less absorption on food, bad appetite, frequent diarrhea, etc. Cardiovascular function will decline with poor blood flow, causing stiffness of limbs and symtoms of headache and dizziness. The middle-aged and the elderly are more likely to suffer from hypertension, coronary heart diseases (CAD) and dementia under this situation accompanied with the symptom of mental deterioration. Lacking exercise can also cause declined immunity, weakening of physical condition and lack of energy. For children, lacking in exercise can lead to short stature with increased risks of injuries, such as ligament sprains during exercise.

（五）锻炼须知

Notes for Exercise

1. 忌在强光下锻炼

Don't Exercise in Bright Light

除游泳外，忌在烈日下锻炼，谨防中暑。夏季阳光中紫外线特别强烈，人体皮肤长时间照射，会发生灼伤。紫外线还会透过皮肤、骨头，辐射到脑膜、视网膜，使大脑和眼球受损伤。

Except for swimming, do not exercise under the scorching sun. Be aware of heat stroke. Ultraviolet rays are particularly strong in summer sunlight, Being exposed under such sunlight for a long period of time can lead to Sunburys. Ultraviolet rays also radiate through the skin and bones to the meninges and retinas, damaging the brain and eyeballs.

2. 忌锻炼时间过长

Don't Exercise for Too Long

一次锻炼时间不宜过长，一般20~30分钟为宜，以免出汗过多，体温上升过高而引起中暑。如果一次锻炼时间较长，可在中间安排1~2次休息。

Exercise time should not be too long in case of heat strokes caused by over-sweating and excessive body temperature. Generally, the recommended time for exercise is about 20 to 30 minutes. If you have to do a long-time exercise, you should have 1 or 2 breaks during the exercise.

3. 忌锻炼后大量饮水

Avoid Drinking Too Much Water after Exercise

锻炼后出汗多，大量饮水会给血液循环系统、消化系统、心脏增加负担。同时，饮水会使出汗增多，盐分则进一步丢失，从而引起痉挛等症状。

Sweating or drinking too much water will add more burden to the blood circulation system, digestive system and heart. Meanwhile, drinking water will lead to more sweating and cause further loss of salt, resulting in cramps and other symptoms.

4. 忌锻炼后立即洗冷水澡

Avoid Taking a Cold Bath Immediately after Exercise

锻炼后体内产热量加快，皮肤毛细血管也大量扩张以便身体散热。突然过冷刺激会使体表已开放的毛孔突然关闭，造成身体内脏器官紊乱，大脑体温调节失常，导致生病。

After exercise, the body heat production increases quickly, and the skin capillaries expand for heat dissipation. Sudden cold stimulation can cause the open pores on the body surface to be suddenly closed, resulting in the body's internal organs disorder. The brain cannot regulate body temperature properly, leading to illness.

5. 忌锻炼后大量吃冷饮

Avoid Having Too Much Cold Drinks after Exercise

锻炼可使大量血液涌向肌肉和体表，而消化系统则处于相对贫血状态。大量的冷饮不仅降低了胃的温度，而且也冲淡了胃液，轻则可引起消化不良，重则会导致急性胃炎。

Exercise causes large amounts of blood to flood into the muscles and body surface, while the digestive system is relatively anemic. Too much cold drinks not only reduce the temperature of the stomach, but also dilute the stomach fluid. In mild cases, it can cause indigestion and in serve cases, it can lead to acute gastritis.

6. 忌锻炼后以体温烘衣

Change Your Clothe after Exercise

有些年轻人认为自己体格健壮而常懒于更换汗衣，这样极易引起风湿病或关节炎。

Some young people might be too lazy to change sweated clothes after exercise. This can easily cause rheumatism or arthritis.

二、心理健康

Mental Health

体育锻炼在很大程度上保证了我们的身体健康，但是在我们有了强健的身体之后，我们也应该把注意力放在心理健康上。什么是心理健康？心理健康是指精神饱满、活动正常、心理素质好。心理健康强调在社交、生产、生活上能与其他人保持较好的沟通或配合，能良好地处理生活中发生的各种情况。

Exercise ensures our physical health to a large extent, but after we have a strong body, we should also focus on mental health. What is mental health? It refers to one's being energetic with normal activities and having good psychological quality. People with good mental health can maintain good connections with others in terms of socialization, routine life and productivity. They have the capacity of dealing with various situations in life in a good and proper way.

（一）影响心理健康的因素

Factors Affecting Mental

能够影响心理健康的因素有很多，但起决定作用的是遗传和环境，尤其是早期的家庭教育。具体的四点如下：

There are many factors that can influence mental health, but the decisive ones are inheritance and external environment, especially the family education at early age. There are four specific points:

①先天遗传的好坏。

The quality of congenital heredity.

②外部刺激的利弊。

Advantages and disadvantages of external stimulus.

③心理素质水平的高低。

The level of psychological quality.

④提供心理健康护理服务的能力。

Ability to provide mental health care services.

（二）维护心理健康的途径

Ways to Maintain Mental Health

①注意优婚优生，避免先天缺陷。

②优化现实环境，减少不良刺激。

③加强心理修养，提高心理素质。

④接受心理教育，学会心理调适。

⑤主动向人求助，及时缓解心病。

Pay attention to eugenics and avoid birth defects.

Optimize the real environment and reduce bad stimuli.

Strengthen psychological cultivation and improve psychological quality.

Receive psychological education and learn psychological adjustment.

Take the initiative to ask people for help; timely relieve sorrow.

（三）心理健康的标准

Mental Health Standards

心理学家将心理健康的标准总结为以下十点：

①有适度的安全感，有自尊心，对自我的成就有价值感。

②适度地自我批评，不过分夸耀自己也不过分苛责自己。

③在日常生活中，具有适度的主动性，不为环境所左右。

④理智、现实、客观，与现实有良好的接触，能容忍生活中挫折的打击。

⑤适度地接受个人的需要，并具有满足此种需要的能力。

⑥有自知之明，了解自己的动机和目的。

⑦能保持人格的完整与和谐，个人的价值观能适应社会的标准，对自己的工作能集中注意力。

⑧有切合实际的生活目标。

⑨具有从经验中学习的能力，能适应环境的需要改变自己。

⑩有良好的人际关系，有爱人的能力和被爱的能力。有个人独立的意见，有判断是非的标准。

Psychologists have set up the criteria for mental health as the following ten points.

1. Have a moderate sense of security, self-esteem, and a sense of value to self-achievement.

2. Have Moderate self-criticism, but do not boast or blame too much.

3. In daily life, be able to take the initiative moderately, not being constrained by the environment.

4. Be rational, realistic, objective, keep good contact with reality and tolerate the frustrations of life.

5. Accept the needs of individuals in a moderate manner and have the ability to meet such needs.

6. Have a self-knowledge, understand their own motives and purposes.

7. Be able to maintain the integrity and harmony of personality, and personal values can adapt to social standards with the ability to concentrate on work.

Have realistic life goals.

Have the ability to learn from experience, and can adapt to the needs of the environment to change their own.

Have good interpersonal relationships, and have the ability to love and the ability to be loved. Have your own independent opinions and the criteria for judging right from wrong.

美国哈佛大学著名精神病学家弗列曼教授认为，在诸多人们患病的原因中，心理因素占了很大比例。世界卫生组织认为心理健康比躯体健康具有更为重要的意义。

Professor Fredman, a famous psychiatrist at Harvard University, believes that "Psychological factors account for a large proportion of people's illness." According to the World Health Organization, mental health is more important than physical health.

三、亚健康

Sub-health

（一）亚健康的定义

Definition of Sub-health

中华中医药学会发布的《亚健康中医临床指南》指出：亚健康指人体处于健康和疾病之间的一种状态。亚健康状态表现为一定时间内的活力降低、功能和适应能力减退的症状，但不符合现代医学有关疾病的临床或亚临床诊断标准。

The Clinical Guidelines for Sub-Health Chinese Medicine published by the Chinese Academy of Traditional Chinese Medicine point out that sub-health refers to a state in which the human body is between health and disease. Sub-healthy people are those who show symptoms of reduced vitality, reduced function and adaptive ability over a certain period of time, but do not meet the clinical or subclinical diagnostic criteria for modern medicine-related diseases.

（二）亚健康的常见症状

Common Symptoms of Sub-Health

亚健康的常见症状有：疲劳、睡眠质量差、失眠、焦虑、情绪波动、脱发以及性欲减退。上述中的任何一条持续发作3个月以上，并且经系统检查排除可能导致上述表现的疾病者，其身体已经处于亚健康状态。

Common symptoms include fatigue, poor sleep quality, insomnia, anxiety, mood swings, hair loss and decreased libido. If any one of these symptoms have persisted for more than 3 months, and you have been systematically screened out for diseases that may cause these symptoms, you are already in a state of sub-health.

四、体育锻炼对心理健康的影响
Effect of Exercise on Mental Health

（一）体育锻炼促进心理健康
Exercise Promotes Mental Health through Exercise

体育锻炼可以促进心理健康，为我们带来很多积极的影响。主要有以下几个方面：

Exercise can promote mental health, and bring us a lot of positive influence, mainly including the following several aspects:

1. 改变情绪状态

Change Your Emotional State

生活在错综复杂的社会中，经常会产生忧愁、紧张、压抑等情绪反应。体育锻炼则可以转移个体不愉快的意识、情绪和行为，使人从烦恼和痛苦中摆脱出来。

Living in the complex society often stimulates the moods of sadness, nervousness, depression, etc. However, exercise can divert one's attention from unpleasant thinking, emotion and behavior as well as any worries or pain.

2. 提高智力

Intelligence Improvement

经常参加体育锻炼也可以提高自己的智力，不仅使锻炼者的注意、记忆、反应、思维和想象能力得到提高，还可以使其情绪稳定、性格开朗、疲劳感下降等。

Regular exercise can also improve our intelligence. It can promote our attention, memory, reaction and imagination ability. Regular exercise can also stabilize emotion, help one to develop an optimistic characteristic, reduce feelings of fatigue, etc.

3. 确立良好的自我概念

Establishing of a Good Self-Concept

自我概念是个体主观对自己的身体、思想和情感的整体评价。如：我是什么人？我主张什么？我喜欢什么？

Self-concept is an individual's subjective evaluation of his or her own body, mind and emotion. Questions like "Who am I?", "What do I believe in?" and "What do I like?" are all a part of self-concept.

4. 培养坚强的意志品质

Developing Strong Character

在体育锻炼中要不断克服困难，也可以把培养起来的坚强意志迁移到日常生活学习中。

In the process of exercise, we can constantly overcome difficulties, thus developing a strong will in daily life.

5. 消除疲劳

Fatigue Elimination

大学生持续紧张的学习压力极易造成身心疲惫和神经衰弱，参加中等强度及以上的体育锻炼可以让身体得到放松。

University students who keep studying intensely can experience exhaustion of both body and mind. Participating in vigorous-intensity physical exercise can help us relax our body.

6. 公认的一种心理治疗方法

A Way of Psychological Treatment

美国的一项调查显示，在1750名心理医生中，有60%的人认为应将体育锻炼作为一种好的方法来消除焦虑症。在大学生中，也有不少人由于学习和其他方面的挫折而引起焦虑症，可以通过体育锻炼来缓解或消除这些心理疾病。

According to a survey in the United States, 60 percent of 1,750 psychiatrists believe that exercise should be used as a way to eliminate anxiety disorders. There are many university students suffering from pressure from study and other setbacks caused by anxiety disorder. For those who are in such condition, they can try to alleviate or eliminate these mental illnesses through exercise.

第二节　体育锻炼与社会健康
Section Two Exercise and Social Health

一、社会健康

Social Health

（一）社会健康的定义与标准

Definition and Standards of Social Health

1. 社会健康的定义

Definition on Social Health

社会健康是一个良性的环境。社会健康也称社会适应性，指个体与他人及社会环境相互作用并具有良好的人际关系和实现社会角色的能力。

By definition, social health is a benign environment. Social health, also known as social adaptability, refers to the ability of individuals to interact with others and social environment and to have good interpersonal relationships with the capability to realize his or her role.

2. 社会健康的标准

Standards for Social Health

社会健康主要由以下标准构成：能接受与他人的差异；与家庭成员和睦相处；有1到2个亲密的朋友；共同工作时，能接受他人的思想与建议；和同性和异性都能够交朋友；当你的观点与大多数人不一致时，你可以继续坚持自己的观点并实践；积极与人交往，人际关系稳定而广泛；在沟通中客观评价别人，取人之长处，弥补自己之短处。

Social health mainly consists of the following standards: to have the ability to accept differences with others; to get along with family members well; to have one or two close friends; When working together, be able to accept the thoughts and suggestions of others; be able to make friends with both genders; when your opinions are at odds with the majority, you can reserve and continue to work; interact with others positively, and have stable and extensive interpersonal relationships; be able to make objective evaluation on other people, and learn from other people.

在这些标准中，可得出的重要的结论是，社会健康需要能够妥善处理人际关系，并在每一段关系中保持健康的互动。

Among these standards, an important conclusion which can be drawn is that social health requires properly handling interpersonal relationships and maintaining healthy interactions in every relationship.

（二）人际关系与社会健康

Relationships and Social Health

社会健康与你和他人的关系紧密相关，人际关系是生活中你与他人、团体交往中形成的关系。良好的关系使你有安全感和归属感，反之，就会有孤独感和退缩感。

Social health is closely related to interpersonal relationship, which is the relationship you form in your life with others and groups. A good interpersonal relationship gives you security and a sense of belonging, while vice versa.

俗话说得好，人类最伟大的成就来自沟通，最大的失败来自不愿意沟通。社会健康水平低会对人们的身心健康产生负面影响，如产生焦虑、抑郁、愤怒等负面情感，最终导致心理疾病。因此，为了保持身心健康，人们需要充足的营养、锻炼、休息等生理上的满足。人们应该如何维持关系？最直接有效的方式是沟通。沟通是人与人之间思想、信仰、观点等方面的交流。沟通帮助我们相互理解、解决冲突、缩短人与人之间的距离。它能够提高自尊，减轻压力，有助于我们身体、精神和社会等方面的自我提升。

As the saying goes, "Man's greatest achievements come from communication, and greatest failures come from the unwillingness to communicate." A low level of social health will have a negative impact on people's physical and mental health, causing as anxiety, depression, anger, etc., eventually leading to psychological disease. Therefore, to maintain physical and mental health, one needs sufficient physiological satisfaction such as nutrition, exercise, rest, etc. The most direct and effective way to maintain and interpersonal relationship is through communication. Communication is the exchange of thoughts, beliefs, and opinions among people. This helps us understand each other, and resolve conflicts, narrowing the gap between people. It improves self-esteem, reduces stress levels, and stimulates physical, mental, and social improvement.

二、体育锻炼对社会健康的作用

The Effect of exercise on Social Health

运动在改善人们的社会健康水平方面起着重要的作用，这是由体育活动的社会特征所决定的。既要相互竞争，也存在交流与合作。同时，这种合作与竞争的行为也会转移到日常生活、学习和工作中。运动对个人的积极影响主要可以分为三个方面：促进人际交往，培养合作精神，形成竞争意识。

Exercise plays an important role in improving people's social health, which is determined by the social characteristics of physical exercise, for in most exercise and physical activities, competition is involved, and thus leads to potential communication and cooperation. Meanwhile, such cooperative and competitive behaviors will also affect daily life, study and work. The positive effects of exercise on individuals can be mainly divided into three aspects: contributing to interpersonal communication; cultivating the spirit of cooperation; forming a sense of competition.

（一）体育锻炼有助于人际交往

Exercise Contributes to Interpersonal Relationship

人际交往是指人们在社会活动中进行交流和情感交流的过程，美国的一项研究表明62%的女性更喜欢和朋友一起锻炼，并认为和同伴一起锻炼是她们坚持锻炼的重要原因之一。

Interpersonal relationship refers to the process in which people carry out communication and emotional exchanges in social activities. A study of the US indicates that 62% of women prefer to exercise with their friends and they believe exercising with friends is an important reason for them to keep exercising.

（二）体育锻炼有助于培养合作精神

Exercise Helps to Cultivate the Spirit of Cooperation

合作能力既是体育活动参与者必备的素质，也是通过体育活动需要发展的一种能力。经常参加体育锻炼，有助于加强合作意识，培养团队精神。

Cooperation ability is not only a necessary quality for participants in sports activities, but also a kind of ability that needs to be developed through sports activities. Regular participation in exercise helps to strengthen the awareness of cooperation and develop team spirit.

（三）体育锻炼有助于形成竞争意识

Exercise Helps to Develop a Sense of Competition

竞争是体育运动的主要特性之一，在运动中，时刻充斥着竞争，既有对自己运动能力的挑战，也有与他人争胜；既有人与人之间的竞争，也有团体与团体之间的竞争。通过竞争有助于培养个体积极进取、顽强拼搏的精神。

Competition is one of the main characteristics of sports. Sports is always full of competition. It not only challenges participants' own athletic skills, but also contains interpersonal competitions as well as team competitions. Through competition, one can develop positive aggressiveness and a strong will.

第三节　体育锻炼与应激
Section Three Exercise and Stress Control

一、应激

Stress

（一）应激的定义与结构

Definition and Structure of Stress

1. 应激的定义

Definition on Stress

应激是个体在"察觉"各种刺激对其生理、心理及社会系统构成威胁时出现的整体现象，所引起的反应可以是适应或适应不良。

Stress is an integral phenomenon that occurs when an individual "perceives" various stimuli and such stimuli threaten his or her physical, psychological and social systems, resulting in a reaction of adaptation or ill-adaptation.

2. 应激的结构

The Structure of Stress

一个完整的应激结构由三个部分构成：应激源，即造成应激或紧张的刺激物；应激本身，即特殊的身心紧张状态；应激反应，即对应激源的生理和心理反应，也称为生理应激与心理应激。

A complete stress structure consists of three parts: the stressor, which refers to the stimulus that causes stress or tension; stress itself, which is a unique status of physical and mental tension; stress response, which is also known as physiological and psychological stress, namely physiological and psychological responses to stress, namely physiological and psychological responses to stressors.

（二）应激对机体的影响

Effects of Stress on Body

应激对人体有着极强的影响。从生物化学角度来说，应激时人体内物质代谢会发生相应的变化，总体的特点是分解增加，合成减少。

Stress can strongly affect the human body. From the perspective of biochemistry, the material metabolism in human body changes correspondingly during stress, with the general characteristics being increased decomposition and decreased synthesis.

1. 心血管系统

Cardiovascular System

应激反应时，引起交感—肾上腺素轴兴奋，儿茶酚胺水平会增高十倍，在早期这一应激反应具有代偿意义，因其会引起心率增高、心排出量增加，小血管收缩，使组织回流量增多，外周阻力升高，有利于维持血压和保证脑、心等重要脏器的血液供应。但是如果应激反应持续存在，大量的内源性去甲肾上腺素和肾上腺素会引起致命性心律失常和心肌坏死，与随后激活的肾素—血管紧张素系统和皮质激素系统会共同造成动—静脉短路开放，血流重新分布，导致内脏供血不足，肾脏和胃肠器官将会容易发生功能障碍。

When experiencing stress response, the sympathetic-adrenaline axis will be stimulated, leading to an increased catecholamine level 10 times more than normal conditions. In the early stage, the stress response can be compensatory, for it result in increased heart rate and cardiac output, and blood vessels will constrict, all of which will increase the back-flowing of the fluid to the body, leading to anincreased peripheral resistance, and thus, creates advantages on maintaining blood pressure and guaranteeing the blood supply for brain, heart and other important organs. But if the stress reaction continues, the excessive amount of endogenous norepinephrine and epinephrine can cause fatal arrhythmia and myocardial necrosis, and then activate the renin-angiotensin system and cortical hormone, commonly leading to hyperactivity-venous short circuit, blood redistribution, causing the insufficient blood supply to organs, and malfunction of the kidney and gastrointestinal organ.

2. 呼吸系统

The Respiratory System

应激状态下，呼吸加快、换气增加，但因应激激素使肺血管收缩，而致肺动脉压力增高、肺间质水肿、通气/血流比例失调，所以有可能引起ARDS（急性呼吸窘迫综合征）。

Under stress state, breathing will accelerate. Stress hormone causes pulmonary vasoconstriction, leading to increased pulmonary artery pressure, pulmonary interstitial edema, and imbalance of ventilation/blood flow, which may cause ARDS (Acute Respiratory Distress Syndrome).

3. 消化系统

Digestive System

所有重大创伤、烧伤、各种休克、心、脑、肾、肝、肺等脏器功能衰竭时，均有可能引起应激性溃疡或急性糜烂性胃炎。

All major trauma, burns, and all kinds of shock, organ failure of heart, brain, kidney, liver, lung, etc., and other organ failure, are likely to cause stress ulcer or acute erosive gastritis.

4. 泌尿系统

Urinary System

在持续而强烈的应激反应情况下，特别是伴有血容量不足、挤压伤致坏死物质大量排出时，肾功能的受损将相当迅速而明显。

Under the condition of continuous and intense stress response, especially accompanied by insufficient blood volume and extrusion injury caused by a large amount of necrotic material excretion, renal function will be damaged rapidy and obviously.

5. 内分泌系统

Endocrine System

由于内脏缺血、缺氧，胰岛对糖的刺激反应降低，胰岛素分泌减少，胰高血糖素分泌增加，组织利用糖明显减少，糖原分解增加。

Due to ischemia and hypoxia in the viscera, the stimulation response of the islets to sugar will decrease with a declined secretion of insulin and an increased secretion of glucagon. Therefore, the utilization of sugar in tissues will decrease significantly, and the decomposition of glycogen will increase.

6. 内环境

Internal Environment

由于血液重新分布，会造成代谢产物积聚和局部酸中毒；除引起内脏器官本身功能障碍之外，还会引起全身内环境紊乱。

The blood redistribution will cause the accumulation of metabolites and local acidosis. which will also cause systemic environmental disorders in addition to the internal organ.

7. 免疫系统

The Immune System

应激状态下，机体分解代谢亢进，合成代谢下降，营养不足，机体呈相对免疫抑制状态。近年来，免疫系统在应激反应中的作用逐渐被重视，并发展成为新型的边缘学科——精神神经免疫学（是心理神经免疫学还是精神神经免疫学）。

Under stress, the organism becomes hyper-catabolic, anabolic, deficient, and relatively immunosuppressed. Nowadays, the function of immune system in stress reaction is greatly valued, which leads to the gradual development into a new subject of Psychoneuroimmunology.

二、应激源

Stressors

（一）应激源的定义

Definition on Stressors

应激源是指能引起全身性适应综合征或局部性适应综合征的各种因素的总称，简单来说，应激源就是引发应激的因素。

Stressors refer to the general term of various factors that can cause General Adaptation Syndrome (GAS) or Local Adaptation syndrome (LAS). In short, stressors are the factors that cause stress.

（二）应激源的类型

Types of Stressors

根据来源不同，应激源可分为以下三类：外部物质环境、个体内环境和心理社会环境。

According to different sources, stressors can be divided into the following three categories: external material environment, internal environment of an individual and psychosocial environment.

1. 外部物质环境

External Material Environment

第一类应激源是外部物质环境。总体来说，外部物质环境包括自然和人为两类因素。属于自然环境变化的有寒冷、酷热、潮湿、强光、雷电、气压等，可以引起冻伤、中暑等反应。属于人为因素的有空气、水、食物及射线、噪音等方面的污染等。

The first type of stressors is the external material environment. Generally speaking, the external material environment includes natural and man-made factors. Changes in the natural environment include cold, heat, humidity, strong light, lightning and air pressure, which can cause reactions such as frostbite and heatstroke. Human factors include pollution on air, water, food, radiation pollution, noise pollution and other pollution, etc.

2. 个体内环境

The Internal Environment of an Individual

第二类应激源是个体的内环境。这里值得注意的是，内、外环境的区分是人为的。内环境的许多问题常来源于外环境，比如营养缺乏、感觉剥夺、刺激过量等。再比如，机体内各种必要物质的平衡失调，如内分泌激素增加，酶和血液成分的改变，既可以是应激源，也可以是应激反应的一个部分。

The second type of stressor is the internal environment of an individual. It is important to note that the distinction between internal and external environments is artificial. Problems in the internal environment are often caused by the external environment, such as lack of nutrition, sensory deprivation, excessive stimulation, etc. Take another example. The imbalance of various essential substances in the body, such as the increase of endocrine hormones, the changes of enzymes and blood composition, can be both the stressor and part of the stress response at the same time.

3. 心理社会环境

Psychosocial Environment

应激源的第三类，是心理社会环境。大量证据表明，心理、社会因素可以引起全身性适应综合征，具有应激性。在现实生活中有许多这样的例子，例如亲人、朋友对我们的影响。尤其是亲人的病故或意外事故常常是重大的应激源，因为在悲伤过程中往往会伴有明显的躯体症状。研究表明，在配偶死亡的这一年中，丧偶者的死亡率比同龄人高出很多倍。

The third type of stressors is the psychosocial environment. A large number of evidences show that psychological and social factors can cause GAS, namely, they have the ability to stress us. There are many examples in our real life.

For instance, the influence of relatives and friends on us, or to be more particular, the death of our loved one or an accident is often a major stressor, as the grieving process is often accompanied by significant physical symptoms. Studies have shown that widowers are much more likely to die during the year of spouse's death than other people of the same age.

根据应激源对人的影响程度，应激又可分为良性应激（生理性应激）和劣性应激（病理性应激）。例如，心理社会因素会引起良性应激，比如中奖、晋升等；也会引起劣性应激，如竞争失败、家庭变故等。从这一点看出，应激对健康具有双重作用。适当的应激可提高机体的适应能力，但过强的应激（不论是良性应激还是劣性应激）使得适应机制失效时会导致机体的功能障碍。

According to the influence degree of stressors on people, stress can be divided into Eustress (physiological stress) and Distress (pathological stress). For example, psychosocial factors can sometimes cause eustress such as winning the lottery, promotion, etc. It can also cause distress, such as failure of competition, misfortune of the family, etc. From this point, it can be seen that stress has a dual effect on health. Appropriate stress can improve the adaptive capacity of the body, but too much stress (whether eustress or distress) will lead to the malfunction of the adaptive mechanism and further lead to the malfunction of our body.

三、应激反应

Stress Response

（一）应激反应的定义

Definition on Stress Response

应激反应其实就是指由各种紧张性刺激物（应激源）引起的个体非特异性反应。

Stress response refers to the individual non-specific response caused by various stressors.

（二）应激反应的类型

Types of Stress Response

应激的具体表现形式因人而异，但归根结底，所有的应激反应都可以划分为两大类：一是活动抑制或完全紊乱，甚至发生感知记忆的错误，表现出不适应的反应，比如目瞪口呆，手忙脚乱，陷入窘境；二是调动各种力量，活动积极，以应对紧急的情况，比如急中生智，行动敏捷，摆脱困境。应激反应包括生理反应和心理反应两大类。范进听说自己中了举人之后的一系列表现就可以理解为应激反应的实例。

Stress response vary from person to person, but generally, all stress responses can be divided into two categories. The first one contains activity inhibition or complete disorder, even the occurrence of perception and memory errors, showing the reaction of maladjustment, such as dumbness, confusion and embarrassment. The second category is to actively respond to the emergency with all available resources and fast reaction as well as wit and wisdom. Stress response includes physiological response and psychological response. Fan Jin's behavior after hearing that he finally succeeded in the exam can be regarded as an example of stress response.

1. 生理反应

Physiological Response

从生物学的角度来说,在应激状态下,生化系统发生激烈变化,肾上腺激素以及各腺体分泌增加,身体活力增强,使整个身体处于充分的动员状态,以应对意外的突变。长期处于应激状态,对人的健康不利,甚至会产生危险。生理反应表现为交感神经兴奋、垂体和肾上腺皮质激素分泌增多、血糖升高、血压上升、心率加快和呼吸加速等。

Under a state of stress, the biochemical system changes violently. Adrenaline and the secretion of glands will increase, and the body becomes more active, leaving the whole body fully in excitement to cope with any unexpected situation. However, to be under state of stress for a long period of time can do harm to people's health and even cause risks to their life. The physiological responses include sympathetic excitation, the increasing of secretion of pituitary and adrenal corticosteroids, increased blood glucose, blood pressure, heart rate and the breath-acceleration, etc.

2. 心理反应

Psychological Response

心理反应包括情绪反应与自我防御反应、应对反应等。应激反应是刺激物同个体自身的身心特性交互作用的结果,不仅仅由刺激物引起,还与个体对应激源的认识、个体处理应激事件的经验等有关。

Psychological response includes emotional responses, self-defense responses and coping responses, etc. Stress response is the result of the interaction between the stimulus and the individual's own physical and mental characteristics. It is not solely caused by the stimulus itself, but is also related to the individual's perspective on the stress source, the individual's experience coping with stress, etc.

(三)应激反应的三个阶段

Three Stages of Stress Response

根据这个过程,科学家将应激反应的全过程进行了分段。1974年加拿大生理学家塞里（G. Selye）的研究表明，应激状态的持续能击溃一个人的生化保护机制，使人的抵抗力降低，容易患身心疾病。他把应激反应称为全身适应综合征，并将其分为三个阶段：

Based on this process, the scientists divided the entire process of stress response into different stages. In 1974, Canadian physiologist G. Selye's research demonstrated that persistence in the state of stress can destroy one's biochemical protection mechanism, which leads to a decline in immunity. People who have long been under stress are more likely to suffer from mental and physical diseases. He called the stress response "general adaptation syndrome" (GAS) and divides it into three stages:

1. 惊觉阶段

Alarm

第一阶段：惊觉阶段，这一阶段肾上腺激素分泌增加，心率加快，体温和肌肉弹性降低，贫血，以及血糖水平和胃酸度暂时性增加，严重的可导致休克。

During the stage of Alarm, the amount of adrenaline secretion will increase with an increased heart rate, decreased body temperature and muscle elasticity, a symptom of anemia and an temporarily increasing of the blood glucose level and stomach acidity. If these symptoms are in severe condition, it can lead to a shock.

2. 阻抗阶段

Resistance

第二阶段：阻抗阶段，此时惊觉阶段症状消失，身体动员许多保护系统去抵抗导致危急的动因，此时全身代谢水平提高，肝脏大量释放血糖。如时间过长，可导致体内血糖的储存大量消耗，以及下丘脑、脑垂体和肾上腺系统活动过度，会给内脏带来物理性损伤，出现胃溃疡、胸腺退化等症状，对我们的身体健康产生影响。

The second stage is Resistance in which the symptoms in the stage of Alarm will disappear. The protective mechanisms of the body will cope with the causes of risks. During this stage, the metabolic level of the whole body will increase, and the liver will release a large amount of blood sugar. However, if this stage lasts for too long, it can lead to the huge consumption on blood sugar as well as the over-activity of hypothalamus, pituitary and adrenal system, which will cause physical damage to the viscera and symptoms such as gastric ulcer, thymus degeneration, etc., eventually endangering our health.

3. 衰竭阶段

Exhaustion

第三阶段：衰竭阶段，这一阶段体内的各种储存几乎耗尽，机体处于危机状态，可导致重病或死亡，十分危险。因此，我们要尽量减少和避免不必要的应激状态，并学会科学地对待应激状态。以高原反应为例。很多人从地势较低的地区去到像青海、西藏之类的高原地区旅游，往往在下飞机时会产生高原反应。人们刚下飞机时体会到的较为剧烈的不适，就是身体处于应激惊觉状态的体现。不过经过一定时间的适应，部分体质较好的人的高原反应会逐渐地消退，这是阻抗阶段的一个表现。但部分人由于体质较差，不能适应高原缺氧的环境，身体长时间处于阻抗阶段，最终进入衰竭阶段，他们的症状会发展成高原水肿或高原脑水肿，这是非常严重和危险的症状。

In the third stage of Exhaustion, energy storage in the body is almost exhausted. The body is in a critical condition which can lead to severe illness or even death. Therefore, we should try to reduce and avoid unnecessary stress and learn to treat stress with appropriate and scientific methods. For example, altitude sickness is something that many people who travel from low-lying areas to plateau areas like Qinghai and Tibet often experience. When experiencing altitude sickness, many people are likely to go through great discomfort as they get off the airplane, which is a sign of the body being in the alarm stage. After a certain period of adaptation, some people with better physical conditions will gradually feel better, which is a sign of the resistance stage. However, due to poor physical condition, some people cannot adapt to the hypoxia on the plateau, and their bodies have been in the resistance stage for too long, which eventually leads to the exhaustion stage. The symptoms will develop into plateau edema or brain edema, which is extremely dangerous.

四、体育锻炼与应激控制
Exercise and Stress Control

（一）体育锻炼控制应激的机理作用
The Mechanism of Controlling Stress through Exercise

据神经内科专家介绍，运动本身可以促进人体的内分泌变化。大脑在运动后会产生一种名为内啡肽的物质，人的心情与大脑内分泌出来的内啡肽相关。运动可以刺激内啡肽的分泌，使内啡肽的分泌增多。内啡肽发挥作用时，会阻碍大脑中与应激有关的化学物的作用，能使人的头脑从担忧以及其他紧张性思维活动中解脱出来。同时，有规律的锻炼会引起身体适应与积极的自我表象，而这两者将提高人对应激的抵抗能力。现代医学证明，正确对待应激事件，利用其积极有利的一面，防止、克服其消极不利的一面，做到乐观、开朗，提高大脑及神经系统的活动力，使机体内各系统的活动协调一致，发挥集中的潜能，有益于身心健康。

According to neurology experts, exercise itself can promote the body's endocrine changes. The brain will produce a substance called endorphin after exercise, and a person's emotion has a great relation to the amount of endorphin. Exercise can stimulate and thus increase the secretion of endorphins. When endorphin is in function, it will block the action of brain chemicals associated with stress, freeing the mind from worries and other stressors. At the same time, regular exercise can lead to better adaptation ability and a positive self-image, both of which increase resistance to stress. Modern medicine has proved that coping with stress appropriately, taking good advantage of its positive side as well as preventing and overcoming its negative side with an optimistic attitude, improving the vitality of the brain and nervous system, coordinating the activities of various systems in the body and realizing collective potential are good for our physical and mental health.

（二）体育锻炼对应激控制的影响
Influence of Exercise on Stress Control

体育锻炼能够降低焦虑水平，但不同的运动类型对应激产生的影响是不同的。因此在了解体育锻炼减少应激的时候，首先应区分短期运动和长期运动对应激反应所产生的不同影响。

Exercise can ease anxiety. Different types of exercise have different effects on stress-coping. Therefore, before learning how exercise can reduce stress, we should first distinguish the effects of short-term exercise and long-term exercise on stress response.

1. 短期运动

Short-term Exercise

短期运动可以转移对应激源的注意力，使人暂时远离一些问题，但这并不意味着逃避问题，在运动之后重新看待问题，情况也许会改善。同时，短期运动可以使人增强自我支配的感觉，从而能够减少应激。比如在体育锻炼中掌握了一定数量和质量的技能之后，这些熟练的技能将会减少和他人进行比赛时的一些生理和心理上的反应。除此之外，短期运动可以通过改善人的心情，减少焦虑和肌肉的紧张。据研究表明，人们在体育锻炼中所产生的良好感觉状态在运动过后将持续6个小时。

In general, short-term exercise can distract you from the stressors and keep you away from the problems which are bothering you. When you look back at these problems after exercising, the situation might improve. At the same time, short-term exercise can make you feel more in control, which can reduce stress. For example, if you acquire a certain amount and quality of skills in exercise, these skills will reduce some of your physical or psychological responses during competitions with others. In addition, short-term exercise can reduce anxiety and muscle tension through mood improvement. According to some studies, people's good mood conducted during exercise can last for 6 hours after exercise.

2. 长期运动

Long-term Exercise

长期有规律的体育锻炼同样可以减少人体的应激反应，比如降低对刺激的觉醒水平，促进应激后机体功能的恢复，改善对某些刺激的心理反应等。不仅如此，长期有规律的体育锻炼还能够减少焦虑和沮丧，预防或者降低抑郁，它是一种有利于降低产生抑郁和焦虑可能性的重要方式。同时，它还可以改善人体的心肺功能、减少体脂，增强机体的适应能力，减少应激。研究表明，和正常人相比，一个具有强健体魄的人在完成同样工作时的心率、血压水平都较低，但他们完成本项任务时所需的基本功能反应时是相等的，只是应激反应减少了。这是因为人体对运动的适应提高了对其他应激的适应能力。

Regular exercise over a long period of time can also reduce stress, lowering levels of arousal to stressors, promoting the recovery of body function after stress and improving the psychological response to certain stimuli. Moreover, regular exercise over a long period of time can reduce anxiety and prevent depression. Meanwhile, it can improve cardiopulmonary function, reduce body fat, enhance the body's ability to adapt and reduce stress. Studies have shown that a physically fit person has lower heart rates, blood pressure, catecholamine levels with fewer stress responses. This is because the body's adaptation to exercise improves its adaption ability to other stresses.

思考

Questions

1. 体育锻炼能在哪些方面影响心理健康？

In what ways can physical exercise affect mental health?

2. 试说明应激源引发应激反应的完整过程。

Try to explain the complete process of stress response caused by stressors.

第四章 健康管理基本操作技能
CHAPTER FOUR BASIC OPERATION SKILLS OF HEALTH MANAGEMENT

我国"十三五"规划提出"大健康"建设，要求群众健康从医疗转向预防为主，不断提高人们自我健康管理意识。健康管理是指一种对个人或人群的健康危险因素进行全面管理的过程。掌握健康管理的基本操作技能可以帮助人们有效开展健康管理工作。本章将对健康管理的基本操作技能进行详细讲解，主要内容包括身体健康状况的测量、身体活动水平的测量及常见疾病的筛查，希望通过本章的学习大家能够更好地了解自身健康状况及身体活动水平，掌握常见慢性病的筛查，以提升自我健康管理综合能力，满足生活中健康管理工作的需要。

The 13rd Five-Year Plan for Economic and Social Development of the People's Republic of China puts forward the construction of "Big Health", which requires public health management to shift from medical treatment to prevention, and to constantly improve public's self-awareness on health management. Health management is a process of comprehensive management ofrisk factorsfor the health of an individual or a certain population. Mastery onbasic skills of health management can effectively improve the self-management of one's health. This chapter willprovide detailed information on the basic skills of health management, including the measurement of health status, the measurement of physical activity level and the screening forcommon diseases. Through this chapter, one can develop a better understanding ofhis or herhealth status and physical activity level and master the screening of common chronic diseases with the intention to improve the comprehensive ability of self-health management and meet the needs of health management in life.

第一节 简单的测量身体健康状况的操作
Section One Operation and Measurement of Health Condition

一、健康状况
Health Status

（一）健康状况的概念

The Concept of Health Status

健康是指一个人在身体、精神和社会等方面都处于良好的状态。传统的健康观是"无病即健康"，现代人的健康观是整体健康，世界卫生组织提出"健康不仅是躯体没有疾病，还要心理健康、社会适应良好和有道德"。

Health refers toa person to be in good physical, mental and social condition. The traditional view onhealth is to be disease-free, while the modern view onhealthfocuses more on an overall health. The World Health Organization puts forward that "health is a state of physical, mental and social well-being and not merely the absence of disease and infirmity".

（二）健康状况的分类与特点

Classification and Characteristics of Health Status

健康状况从医学角度而言分3类，分别为健康状态、亚健康状态以及不健康状态。

From the medical perspective, health status can be divided into three categories: healthy, sub-healthy and unhealthy

1.健康状态

Health Status

健康状态指人的主要系统、器官功能正常、无疾病、体质状况和体力水平等指标正常。

Health status usuallyrefers to the good function of one's bodily systems and organs, disease-free, and the normality of physical fitness indicators.

2.亚健康状态

Sub-health Status

亚健康状态是指人体处于健康与疾病之间的临界状态，虽然各类检验结果均为正常，但人体仍有不适感。

Sub-health status refers to the critical state between health and diseasewithdiscomfort of the body despite all medical test results being normal.

3.不健康状态

Unhealthy Status

不健康状态是指患有疾病。

The unhealthy status refers to one with illness.

二、健康状况的常用测量操作技术

Common Techniques for Measuring Health Status

健康状况测量常用操作技术主要包括：身高、体重、头围、腰围、血压等的测量。

Common techniques for health status measurements include the following indicators: height, weight, head circumference, waist circumference, blood pressure, etc.

（一）身高测量

Height

身高测量，多以厘米（cm）为单位，精确到0.1厘米。不同群体测量身高的操作方法不尽相同。

Height is mostly measured in centimeters(cm)with an accuracyofcentimeters.

The measurement for height will differ for various groups of people.

1. 针对3岁及以上的儿童和成人

For Children Over 3 Years Old and Adults

测量前校正立柱与踏板垂直，活动自如；测量时需要脱去鞋、帽等服饰，立正、收腹、两臂下垂保持正确的体态。

Before measuring, the column and the peddle should be adjusted into a vertical position and can be moved freely. When measuring, footwear and headwear should be removed. The subject should stand straight and tighten the abdomen with both arms hanging downwards.

2. 针对3岁以下的儿童

For Children Under 3 Years Old

测量时要将测量板平放；被测量者处于仰卧位；脱去鞋、帽、厚衣服等；保持被测量者的头部固定；贴紧测量板，双腿伸直。

When measuring, the measuring plate should be laid flat. The subject should be in the supine position. Footwear and headwear should be removed as well as any thick wearing. The subject's head should remain fixed and be kept close to the measuring pad with legs straightened.

（二）体重测量

Weight

体重测量，多以千克（kg）为单位，精确到0.1千克。针对不同群体测量的单位不尽相同。

Weight is usually measured in kilograms(kg) with an accuracy of 0.1 kg. Different measuring units are used for different populations.

1. 针对3岁及以上的儿童和成人

For Children Over 3 Years Old and Adults

针对3岁及以上的儿童和成人多以千克作为单位，精确到0.1千克。在测量前要检查零点校准仪器，把误差控制在0.1千克内。被测量者需要脱鞋、帽子，还有外套等。

For adults and children over 3 years old, the measuring unit used is kilogramwith an accuracy of 0.1kg. A zero calibration should be conducted for the measuring instrument before the measuring to control the error within 0.1 kg. The subjects need to take off footwear and headwear as well as coats if wearing.

2.针对3岁以下儿童

For Children Under 3 Years Old

针对3岁以下的儿童要将读数记录到0.01千克。

The result of a child under three years old should be accurate to 0.01 kilogram when recording.

3.测量影响因素及注意事项

Influential Factors and Precautions

（1）影响因素

Influencing Factors

测量结果受到不同因素的影响，同一个人的体重在一天之内的不同时刻可以相差1千克以上，比如吃饭或喝水前后、睡觉前后、大小便前后所称量的体重就会有所差异，但这种差异只在一定范围内有规律地上下波动，属于一种十分正常的现象。

The results may be affected by different factors. The weight of a same person can differ by more than 1kg at different times of aday. For example, the weight measured before and after eating, drinking, sleeping, urinating or defecating may vary. However, this difference only fluctuates regularly within a certain range, which is anormal phenomenon.

（2）注意事项

Precautions

为了避免测量误差，在测量体重时，应选择在每日、每周或每月的相同时间以及相似条件下进行，最好选择在清晨起床排便后、早餐前，或沐浴后赤脚穿内衣裤时进行称量，并记录下当时的实际体重，然后再和以往的记录进行比较。

In order to avoid errors, weight should be measured at the same time every day, every week or every month under similar conditions. It is better to weigh after getting up in the morning and defecating, before breakfast, or when wearing underwear after bathing. Record the actual weight at that time, and then compare with the previous records.

（三）头围测量

Head Circumference

头围测量，多以厘米（cm）为单位，精确到0.1厘米。测量3岁以下儿童的头围时，软尺起于右侧眉弓上缘，从头右侧经枕骨粗隆最高处回到起点，贴紧皮肤。正常的成年人也是如此测量，长发者软尺经过处上下分开。

Head circumference should be measured in centimeter (cm) with an accuracy of 0.1 cm. For children under 3 years of age, the tape measure should circle the head from the right and pass through the highest point of the occipital bone with the upper edge of the right eyebrow arch as a starting point. When measuring, thetape measure should keep close to the skin. Adults can also be measured in such way and for those long hear, their hair should be divided into two parts by the tape measure.

（四）腰围测量

Waist Circumference

腰围测量，多以厘米（cm）为单位，精确到0.1厘米。不同群体测量腰围的操作要求不尽相同。

Waist circumferenceis usually measured in centimeter (cm) with an accuracy of 0.1 cm. Different measuring standards are required for different populations.

1.针对15岁及以上的被测量者

For Participants Aged 15 and Above

15岁及以上被测量者在测量时要注意测量时的姿势。身体直立，腹部放松，软尺贴近皮肤，保持呼吸平静。可以测量两次，取平均值作为结果。

For thoseaged 15 and above,body posesareof great importance when being measured. The subject should stand straight and relax the abdomen, with calm breaths. The tape measure should keep close to the skin.The result can be an averaged number of two measuring.

2.针对15岁以下的被测量者

For Participants Under 15 Years Old

由于15岁以下的被测量者身体还处于发育状态,故对于腰围没有严格的测量要求。

Since the bodies of the participants under 15 years old arestill in a developing state, there is no strict measurement requirement for waist circumference.

(五)血压测量

Measurement of Blood Pressure

血液在血管内流动时,对血管壁的侧压力称为血压。血压通常指动脉血压或体循环血压,是重要的生命体征。血压测量是评估血压水平、诊断高血压及观察降压疗效的主要手段,准确地测量血压是基层开展高血压管理的基础。正常值参考范围:收缩压90~140毫米汞柱;舒张压60~90毫米汞柱;脉压30~40毫米汞柱。血压测量的类型包括,诊所偶测血压、自我测量血压和动态血压监测。

As blood flows through a vessel, the lateral pressure on the vessel wall becomes blood pressure. Blood pressure usually refers to arterial blood pressure or systemic blood pressure, and is a vital sign of great importance. Blood pressure can be an indicator to evaluate blood pressure level, diagnose hypertension and observe antihypertensive effect.The accurate blood pressure measurement is the basis to conduct hypertension control on primary level. The range of normal value is90 ~ 140mmHg for systolic blood pressure (SBP), 60~90mmHgfor diastolic blood pressure (DBP), and30 ~ 40mmHg forpulse pressure. Types of blood pressure measurements include clinical casual blood pressure, self-measured blood pressure and dynamic blood pressure monitoring.

1.诊所偶测血压

Clinical Casual Blood Pressure

进行诊所偶测血压时,首先静息5分钟,测前30分钟禁烟、咖啡,排空膀胱。保持坐位,露右上臂,肘部与心脏平齐,特殊情况可取站立位或卧位。

In the condition of the clinical casual blood pressure test, no smoking or coffee is allow and the bladder should be emptied 30 minutes before the testing. Then take a 5-mintue rest. During the testing, keep seatedand expose the right upper arm with the elbow at the samelevel of your heart. Standing or decubitus position can be considered under special circumstances.

2.自我测量血压

Self-measured Blood Pressure

自测血压时，方法同诊所偶测血压，自测时以2次读数的平均值计数，记录测量日期、时间、地点及活动情况。可使用符合国际标准（BHS和AAMI）的上臂全自动或半自动电子血压仪。半自动电子血压仪需要手动按压气囊充气，全自动的只需按下开关就能自动加压。

Self-measured blood pressure uses the same method as the clinical casual blood pressure. During the self-measured blood pressure, an averaged reading of two measuring will be recorded along with the date, time, place and activity of the measurement. Automatic or semi-automatic electronic upper arm blood pressure gauges conforming to international standards (BHS and AAMI) can be used. The semi-automatic electronic blood pressure meter needs users to manually press the air bag to inflate, while the automatic blood pressure meter can automatically pressurize by pressing the switch.

3.动态血压监测

Dynamic Blood Pressure Monitoring

动态血压监测，指使用符合国际标准（BHS和AAMI）的监测仪，在日常生活状态下，测压间隔时间为15~30分钟，白天与夜间测压间隔时间相同，监测24小时。提供白天、夜晚各时间段血压均值的离散情况，动态观察血压的变化，及昼夜血压差异，估计靶器官损害疾病。

Dynamic blood pressure monitoring refers to the monitoring which use monitors in accordance with international standards (BHS and AAMI). In daily life, the interval time of pressure measurement is 15~30minutes, daytime and night pressure measurement interval time is the same, monitoring 24 hours. Dispersed mean values of blood pressure at 24 hours, in the day and at night were provided to dynamically observe the changes of blood pressure and the differences between day and night blood pressure to estimate target organ damage diseases.

4. 测量注意事项

Precautions for Measurement

肥胖者和儿童进行测量时，要注意袖带是否合适。根据柯氏音血压测量方法，血压测量分为5个阶段，第一时相时，仪器读取收缩压，第五时相时，读舒张压。儿童、妊娠妇女以及心脏疾病的患者在第四时相时进行读取。每隔2分钟重测一次，取平均值作为最后结果。当选用全自动或半自动血压仪的时候，最后仪器会按上述原则自动显示出被测者的脉搏值和血压值。

When measuring obese individualand children, Attention should be focused on whether the cuffs fit the subject. According to Korotkoff's sounds electronic measuring method, blood pressure measurement can bedivided into 5 stages. In the first stage, the systolic pressure will be recorded. In the fifth stage, the diastolic pressurewill be measured. Children, the pregnant, and patients with heart disease areread during the fourth stage. When measuring, the measurement will be repeated every two minutes and an averaged reading of all measurements will be considered as the final. Automatic andsemi-automatic blood pressure gauges will automatically display the pulse and blood pressure of the subject according to the principles above.

三、健康状况测量指标及评价

Measurement Indicators and Evaluation of Health Status

（一）健康状况测量指标的功能及分类

Function and Classification of Health Status Indicator

1. 测量指标的功能

Function of Measurement Indicator

测量指标能够反映出所测事物的属性和特征，帮助人们深入了解被测事物的实质。

Measurement indicator can reflect the attributes and characteristics of the subject with the initial purpose to assist other gain further information on the subject.

2. 测量指标的分类

Classification of Measurement Indicator

从健康状况的概念出发，判断被测的健康状况并分析评价其健康水平，常用以下健康指标：

To determine the health status ofa subjectas well as to analyze and to evaluate his or her physicalhealth level, the following health indicators are commonly used:

（1）人口学指标

Demographic Indicator

该指标包括总出生率、总死亡率、婴儿死亡率、5岁以下儿童死亡率、人口平均期望寿命等。

Demographic indicators include total birth rate, total mortality rate, infant mortality rate, mortality rate of children under 5, and average life expectancy of the population, etc.

（2）生长发育指标

Growth Indicator

该指标针对0-14岁或0-17岁年龄段的儿童、青少年生长发育状况，包括其被测者的形态、功能、肌力、智能、性成熟。

Growth indicator is designed to monitorfor the physical developmentof children and adolescents aged from 0 to 14 or from 0 to 17, including the physical shape, body function, strength, intelligence and sexual maturity.

（3）疾病、伤残指标

Disease and Disability Indicator

该指标包括传染病和寄生虫的发病率、职业病和职业性外伤的发病率、慢性病的患病率、因病或因伤致残的残疾率。

Disease and Disability Indicators include the incidence of infectious diseases and parasites, the incidence of occupational diseases and occupational trauma, the incidence of chronic diseases, and the rate of disability due to injury.

（4）社会心理卫生状况指标

Social and Mental Health Indicator

该指标包括青少年犯罪率、青少年吸烟率、自杀发生率和离婚率等。

Physiological Health Indicator includephysical shape, body function, sexual maturity, nutrition status, medical history and family history of illness.

（5）生理健康状况指标

Physiological Health Indicator

该指标包括形态、功能、性成熟、营养状况、疾病史和疾病家族史。

This indicator includes morphology, function, sexual maturity, nutritional status, medical history and family history of illness.

（6）心理健康指标

Mental Health Indicator

该指标包括人格、智力、情感。

Mental Health Indicatorsincludes personality, intelligence and emotion.

（7）社会特征指标

Social Characteristics Indicator

该指标包括行为模式、生活方式、人际关系、个人经济、政治地位、个人经历。

Social Characteristics Indicators include behavior pattern, lifestyle, interpersonal relationship, personal finance, political status and personal experience.

（二）个体健康状况评价

Individual Health Evaluation

1. 单个指标评价

Evaluation of Individual Indicator

标准体重（kg）：男性＝身高(cm)－105；

女性＝身高（cm）－100

理想体重（kg）：男性＝身高（cm）－105－（身高－152）×2/5；

女性＝身高（cm）－100－（身高－152）×2/5

超重：超过标准体重10%为偏重，超过20%为肥胖

Standard weight(kg): male=height(cm)−105;

Female=height(cm)−100

Ideal weight(kg): male=height(cm)−105−(height−152)×2/5;

Female=Height(cm)−100−(Height−152)×2/5

Overweight: 10% over the standard body weight is overweight, over 20% is obese.

2. 综合评价

Comprehensive Evaluation

利用身体质量指数［（BMI）=体重（kg）/身高^2（m）］综合评价身高、体重测量指标，此身体质量指数适用于除孕妇和肌肉强健人群之外所有18至65岁的人群。由于不同人种体质上的差别，分为WHO标准、亚洲标准和中国参考标准，可根据个人的情况，进行自我评价。

Body Mass Index [BMI: weight(kg)/height2 (m)] isused to evaluate height and weight measures. BMI isapplicable to all people aged from 18 to 65 years except pregnant women and those with strong muscles. Three standards are developed for BMI measurement according to the differences between races and populations, including WHO standard, Asian Standard and Chinese Standard.

第二节　身体活动水平的测量
Section Two Measurement of Activity

在日常的运动活动中，利用代谢当量和自觉运动强度调控运动时强度，并且利用量表测量和日志记录的方法测量和计算运动能量的消耗。

In daily exercise activities, we can use metabolic equivalent and the rating of perceived exertion (RPE) to regulate exercise intensity, and use scale measurement and log recording to measure and calculate exercise energy consumption.

一、日常活动水平的测量
Measures for Aerobic and Endurance Exercise

日常活动的水平测量包括有氧和耐力运动量的测量，肌肉力量和耐力的测量。

The measurement of daily activities levels includes measures foraerobic and endurance exercise and measures formuscle strength and endurance.

（一）有氧和耐力运动量的测量途径

Measurement of Aerobic and Endurance Exercise

1. 心率测量

Heart Rate

（1）心率及其相关定义

Heart Rate and Definitions

心率是指正常人安静状态下每分钟心跳的次数，也叫安静心率，一般为60-100次/分钟，可因年龄、性别或其他生理因素产生个体差异。一般来说，年龄越小，心率越快，老年人心跳比年轻人慢，女性的心率比同龄男性快，这些都是正常的生理现象。安静状态下，成人正常心率为60~100次/分钟，理想心率应为55-70次/分钟（运动员的心率较普通成人偏慢，一般为50次/分钟左右）。心率在运动过程中很大程度上是运动强度的数值反馈，对于心率进行测量能够准确了解自身运动的强度。

Heart rate refers to a person' sheart beats per minute under calm situation, also called quiet heart rate. Normally, a person's heart rate should be at 60~100 beats per minute. However, age, gender or other physical factors can cause difference on heart rate between different individuals. In general, a person' sheart rate will gradually drop as he or she ages. The heart rate of women is faster than aman atthe same age. These are all normal physiological phenomena. Under the calmsituation, the normal heart rate of adults is 60~100 beats/min, and the ideal heart rate should be 55~70 beats/min (the heart rate of athletes is slower than that of ordinary adults, usually about 50 beats/min). Heart rate is, to a large extent, the numerical feedback of exercise intensity in the process of exercise and measuring heart rate can help one accurately understand the intensity of exercise.

（2）心率的测量的内容与方法

Content and Method of Heart Rate Measurement

心率的测量内容包括目标心率、最大心率和最大储备心率。运动心率与运动强度的关系为大强度运动，是最大心率的80%以上；中等强度运动，是最大心率的60%~80%；低强度运动，是最大心率的60%以下。通常在快速步行10分钟后，即刻进行心率测试。

Heart rate measurements include target heart rate, maximum heart rate and maximum reserve heart rate. The relationship between heart rate and exercise intensity is as follows. High intensity exercise can cause heart rate rising tomore than 80% of the maximum heart rate, Moderate intensity exercise60 to 80 percent of maximum heart rate, and low intensity exercise less than 60% of maximum heart rate. A heart rate test is usually conducted immediately after a brisk walk of 10 minutes.

①目标心率（Target Heart Rate），指用心率监测运动强度，可以通过触摸颈动脉或四肢动脉直接进行测量，运动心率＝运动时每分钟的脉搏数，测量10秒，乘以6；也可采用有线和无线仪器设备监测心率。

The Target Heart Rate refers to the heart rate whichcan used to monitor the exercise intensity. It can be measured directly through the pulse of your carotid or extremity arteries. Target Heart Rate =10s' pulse number per minute during exercise, measuring 10s by 6. Certain devices can also be used to monitor the heart rate.

②最大心率（MHR），可通过逐级递增试验测定，也可按年龄进行计算，最大心率（次/分钟）＝220（次/分钟）－年龄

Maximum heart rate(MHR) can be calculatedthrough anIncremental Step Test maximum or directly through a formula based on age which is shown as followed:

Maximum Heart Rate(beats/minute)=220(beats/min)－age

③最大储备心率（MHRRmax）（次/分钟）＝最大心率（次/分钟）－安静心率（次/分钟）

Maximum Heart Rate Reserve(MHRR)(beats/min) = Maximum heart rate(beats/min) - Resting Heart Rate(beats/min)

（3）不同心率区间的作用

The Role of Different Heart Rate Zones

当运动强度达到50%~60%最大心率时，运动类型为适应性热身，对于机体具有恢复机能的功能，新陈代谢以脂肪为主，建议维持的活动时间是20~40分钟；当运动强度达到60%~70%最大心率时，运动类型为有氧运动，对于进行减肥具有良好效果，主要代谢以脂肪和少部分碳水化合物，建议维持的活动时间是40~80分钟；当运动强度达到70%至80%的最大心率，运动类型为有氧运动，有助于提高运动者的运动状态并提高心肺能力，代谢少部分脂肪，主要以碳水化合物的代谢形式，建议维持活动时间为10~40分钟；当运动强度达到80%~90%的最大心率，该阶段运动类型处于有氧与无氧的临界，其主要代谢机体碳水化合物以及糖类，有助于提高运动者的运动绩效、增肌、增强集体乳酸忍耐度，建议维持运动时间为2~10分钟；当运动强度增加到90%的最大心率时，其运动类型为无氧运动，主要代谢机体糖类，能够让速度最大限度上进行提高、增肌以及增进心肺能力，同时该强度下建议运动时间维持少于5分钟。

When the exercise intensity reaches 50% to 60% of the maximum heart rate, the exercise type is a warm-up, serving as therestoration for body function, consuming mainly fat, with a recommended exercise time of 20 to 40 minutes. When the intensity of exercise reaches 60% to 70% of the maximum heart rate,it can be considered as an aerobic exercise whichis efficient on weight loss. Themetabolismof fat and a small amountof carbohydrate is dominant. The recommended exercise timeis 40~80 minutes. When the intensity of exercise reaches 70% to 80% of the maximum heart rate, the type of exercise is aerobic exercise, which is helpful to improve the exercise state and improve the cardiopulmonary capacity. The metabolism of carbohydrate is dominant with a small amount of fat. For this exercise type, recommended duration is 10~40 minutes. When the exercise intensity reaches 80% to 90% of the maximum heart rate, the type of exercise in this stage is at the threshold of aerobic and anaerobic.

Carbohydrates and sugars in the body is mainly metabolize, which is helpful to improve the exercise performance of the exercisers, build muscle and enhance collective lactate tolerance. It is recommended to maintain suchexercise for 2~10 minutes. When the exercise intensity increases to 90% of the maximum heart rate, the exercise type is an anaerobic exercise, which mainly metabolizes sugars in the body and can maximize the consuming speed. This type of exercise is good for muscle building andcardiopulmonary capacity improving.It is recommended less than 5 minutes for such exercise intensity.

（4）最适宜运动心率的计算方法与注意事项

Calculation Method and Precautions of Optimal Exercise Heart Rate

最适宜运动的心率，即运动靶心率，其计算公式为：运动靶心率＝心率储备×（60%－80%）+安静心率。例如某人40岁，安静时的心率为每分钟80次。按照上述方法计算：最大心率220bpm－40bpm＝180bpm；心率储备180bpm-80bpm＝100bpm；最适宜的运动心率100bpm×60%＝60bpm，100bpm×80%＝80bpm，80bpm+60＝140bpm，80bpm+80＝160bpm，其最适宜的运动心率应在140~160次/分钟之间，进行运动的过程中其运动强度要控制好，让心率在140~160次/分钟之间最合适，过低则运动效果达不到，过高则对身体压力较大，产生负面效果。

The most suitable heart rate for exercise is the target rate for exercise. Its calculation formula is as follows: Target Rate for Exercise = Heart Rate reservedx 60%~80%+Resting Heart Rate. For example, a personis 40 years old and his or her resting heart rate is 80 beats/min. According to this formula, this person's target rate for exercise can be calculated as the following steps: Maximum heart rate: 220bpm—40=180bpm; HeartRate Reserved: 180bpm— 80 =100bpm. Target Heart Rate forExercise:100bpmx60%=60bpm, 100bpmx80%=80bpm; 80bpm + 60bpm=140bpm; 80bpm + 80bpm=160bpm. The target heart rate forexercise should be between 140~160 times/minute. If it is too low, the exercise will be less effective and onceit is too high, exercise might cause negative effects on body.

确定靶心率还应该根据具体情况，不同时期的健康状态、环境、季节、心情等对选择运动量会产生一定的影响。感冒或患其他急性病期间、处于闷热的气候、暴晒的环境或大悲大喜等时候，运动强度和运动时间均要相应降低，心率指标亦相应降低，以保证安全。相反，随着有氧运动能力的提高，靶心率就可以作相应的提高，以增强健身效果。

The target heart rate should also be flexible according to specific situations. The health status, environment, season, mood and other factors can affect the selection of exercise intensity. When suffering from a cold or other acute diseases, in sultry climate or insolate environment orexperiencing great mood swings, exerciseintensity and exercisetimeshould be relatively reduced as well asrelevant heart rate index in order to ensure safety. On the contrary, with the improvement of aerobic exercise ability, the target heart rate can be improved accordingly to enhance the fitness effect.

2.代谢当量（METs）

Metabolic Equivalents(METs)

（1）代谢当量的定义

Definition

代谢当量是以安静且坐位时的能量消耗为基础，表达各种活动时相对能量代谢水平的常用指标。1MET被定义为每公斤体重每分钟消耗3.5毫升氧气，大概相当于一个人在安静状态下坐着，没有任何活动的，每分钟氧气消耗量。一个5MET的活动表示运动时氧气的消耗量是安静状态时的5倍。

Metabolic equivalent is a commonly used index to express the relative energy metabolism level of various activities based on the energy consumption. 1 MET is defined as 3.5 milliliters of oxygenconsumption per minute per kilogram of body weight, which is roughly equivalent to the consumption of oxygen per minute by a person sitting quietly without any activity. A 5 METS exercise means that oxygen consumption during exercise is five times higher than at rest.

（2）代谢当量的测量内容与方法

Measurement Content and Method of Metabolic Equivalent

美国运动医学会（American College of Sports Medicine, ACSM）设计了用于计算走路、跑步、固定自行车、台阶的总氧气消耗量（Gross VO$_2$）的代谢当量公式。由于没有考虑到年龄、性别、运动技巧和体格大小对于这些运动类型的能量消耗的影响，因此这些公式只是相对精确地估算运动时总氧气消耗量（Gross VO$_2$）。

每次运动总氧气消耗量（Gross VO$_2$）＝3.5+0.2×（速度）+0.9×（速度）×（坡度百分比）

总代谢当量（Gross METs）＝总氧气消耗量（Gross VO$_2$）÷3.5毫升/千克/分钟

净代谢当量（Net METs）＝总代谢当量（Gross METs）－1安静时代谢当量（MET）

The American College of Sports Medicine (ACSM) has developed a metabolic equivalent formula for calculating the Gross VO$_2$ of walking, running, stationary cycling and stairs-walking. Since neglecting how age, gender, exercise skills and physical shape can affectthe energy consumptionof exercise, these formulas only provide relatively accurate estimates of Gross VO2 during exercise.

Total oxygen consumption per exercise Gross VO$_2$＝3.5+0.2×(speed)+0.9×(speed)×(slope percentage)

Gross METs＝ Gross VO$_2$÷3.5ml/kg/min

Net METs＝Gross METs －1MET

3.自觉运动强度（RPE）

Rating of Perceived Exertion(RPE)

（1）自觉运动强度的定义

Definition

运动自觉强度RPE（Rating of Perceived Exertion），指将费力程度数值化，并且作为运动强度指标的方法。任何运动都可以使用运动自觉强度衡量运动强度是否适中，许多职业运动员更以运动自觉强度替代心跳率计算。使用运动自觉强度时，注意不要让心理因素影响判断，有些运动员会因心理因素而低估强度导致过量训练，如此RPE量表便失去了效用。

Rating of Perceived Exertion is a method of quantifying perceived exertion intoan index to evaluateexercise intensity. RPE can be used to evaluate the intensity ofall exercise.Many professional athletes use RPE to evaluate exercise intensity instead of heart rate. When using the RPE, it should be noted that psychological factors should not affect the judgment on RPE. Some athletes may underestimate the RPE due to psychological factors, leading to overtraining. In such circumstance, RPE can lose its effectiveness.

（2）自觉运动强度的测量内容及方法

Method for Measurement of RPE

运动生理学家和医生们已广泛应用"运动自觉量表"，受测者可以立即描述出运动时主观感觉的劳累程度。体能教练在指导学员时也可以采用这个方法，可以单独使用，也可以和测量心率的方法同时使用，以监测运动强度是否适当。此次我们来介绍下柏格自觉吃力程度量表（见下表），其从0至10以数字大小表示强度，内容包括：

Rating Scaleof Perceived Exertion is widely used by exercise physiologists and doctors, which allows participants to immediately describe how subjectively tired they areduring exercise. Physical fitness trainers can also use this method when working with their trainees.RSPE can be used alone or in conjunction with heart rate measurements to monitor whether the intensity of activity is appropriate. Here we will introduce Borg Rating Scale of Perceived Exertion, which is used to indicate the exercise intensity from the scale of 0 to 10.

柏格自觉吃力程度量表

Borg Rating Scale of Perceived Exertion

等级Level	自感强度Perception	等量典型运动 Equivalent Typical Exercise
0	没感觉No Feeling	休息Resting
1	很弱Very Weak	阅读Reading
2	弱Weak	穿衣Dressing
3	温和Gentle	室内慢走Indoor Walking
4	稍强Slightly Stronger	室外慢走WOutdoorWalking
5	强Strong	走进商店Walking ina Department Store
6	中强Moderately Strong	赶着赴约Rush to a Date
7	很强Very Strong	剧烈运动Strenuous Exercise
8	非常强Vigorous Strong	激烈运动Vigorous Exercise
9	超强Super Strong	极剧烈运动Most Strenuous Exercise
10	极强Extremely Strong	精疲力竭Complete Exhaustion

0级——没什么感觉

Level 0- No Feeling

这是你在休息时的感觉，你丝毫不觉疲惫，你的呼吸完全平缓，在整个运动期间你完全不会有此感觉。

This is how you feel when you are resting, not tired at all. Your breathing is completely smooth and will not feel this during the whole exercise.

1级——很弱

Level 1- Very Weak

这是你在桌前工作或阅读时的感觉，你丝毫不觉疲惫，而且呼吸平缓。

This is how you feel when you work or read at the desk with a calm breathing.

2级——弱

Level 2- Weak

这是你在穿衣服时可能出现的感觉，你稍感疲惫或毫无疲惫感，你的呼吸平缓，运动时很少会体验到这种程度的感觉。

This is the sensation that you may experience when you are wearing clothes. You might feel a little tired or not tired at all. Your breathing is calm. You can seldom experience such perception during exercise.

3级——温和

Level 3- Gentle

这是你慢慢走过房间打开电视机时可能出现的感觉，你稍感疲惫，你可能轻微地察觉到你的呼吸，但气息缓慢而自然，在运动过程初期你可能会有此感觉。

This is the sensation you may experience when you slowly walk through the room and turn on the TV. You might be a little tired, and you might be slightly aware of your breathing, but the breath is slow and natural. You may feel this in the early exercise process.

4级——稍强

Level 4- Slightly Strong

这是你在户外缓慢步行时可能产生的感觉，你感到轻微疲惫，呼吸微微上扬但依然自在。在热身的初期阶段可能会有此感觉。

This is the sensation that you may have when you are walking slowly outdoors. You might slightlyfeel tired with aslightly intensifiedbreathing,but still feel comfortable. This feeling might appear in the early stages of warming up.

5级——强

Level 5- Strong

这是你轻快地走向商店时可能出现的感觉，你感到轻微的疲惫，你察觉到自己的呼吸，气息比第4级还急促一些，你在热身结尾时会有此感觉。

This is the sensation that may occur when you walk briskly to the store. You feel slightly tired. You perceive your breathing. The breath is faster than that of level 4. You will feel this at the end of the warm-up.

6级——中强

Level 6- Moderately Strong

这是你约会迟到急忙赶去时可能出现的感觉，你感到疲惫，但你知道你可以维持这样的步调，你呼吸急促，而且可以察觉得到。从暖身转向运动阶段的期间，以及在学习如何达到第7级和第8级的初期里，你都可能有此感觉。

This is the feeling that you mightexperience when you are rushing to a late date. You will feel tired, but you will have no trouble to maintain yourpace. You might be slightlyout of breath, and you can realize such shor of breath. You may feel this during the transition from warm-up to exercise, and during the early stages of learning how to reach levels 7 and 8.

7级——很强

Level 7- Very Strong

这是你激烈运动时可能出现的感觉，你势必感到疲惫，但你可以确定自己可以维持到运动结束，你绝对会感觉到你的呼吸急促，你可以与人对话，但你可能宁愿不说话，这是你维持运动训练的底线。

This is the feeling that you may experience when you are exercise intensely. Tireness will definitely be realized, but you can also be sure that you can finish this period of exercise. A rapid breathing can be easily realized by you. You can talk people thoughyou mightprefer not to.This is your threshold to decide whether you will keep exercising.

8级——非常强

Level 8- Vigorous Strong

这是你做非常剧烈的运动时可能出现的感觉，你势必感到极度疲惫，而你认为自己可以维持这样的步调直到运动结束，只是你无法百分之百地确定。你的呼吸非常急促，你还是可以与人对话，但你不想这么做。这个阶段只适用于你已能自在地达到第7级，并准备好做更激烈的训练。这一级会让你产生迅速的效果，但你必须学习如何维持，对许多人而言，这么剧烈的运动不容易做到。

This is the feeling that you may experience when you are do highlyintensiveexercise. You will be extremely tired, and you think you can maintain suchpace to finish the exercise without a100% sure. You are breathing rapidly.You can still talk to people, but you don't want to. This stage is only suitable for you when you can reach level 7 comfortably and are ready to do more intensive training. This level will allow you to produce some rapid improvements on your exercise ability, but you must learn how to maintain it. For many people, such strenuous exercise is hard to keep up.

9级——超强

Level 9- Super Strong

这是极度剧烈运动下所出现的感觉，你势必体验到极度的疲惫，如果你自问是否能持续到运动结束，你的答案可能是否定的。你的呼吸非常吃力，而且无法与人交谈，你可能在试图达到第8级的片刻，会有此感觉。这是许多专业运动员训练的级数，对他们而言，要达到这个级数也非常困难，你的例行运动不应该达到第9级，而当你达到第9级时，你应该让自己慢下来。

This is the sensation that appears under extreme strenuous exercise. Extreme fatigue is inevitable. You will consider yourself not able to keep in pace to finish the exercise. You will experience a hard time on breathing and you will be unable to speak to others. You may experience this when you are trying to reach level 8 of exercise. This is the level that many professional athletes training under.For them, it is also very difficult to reach this level. Your routine exercise should not reach level 9 and when you reach level 9, you should ease on your exercise.

10级——极强

Level 10- Extremely Strong

你不应该经历第10级，在这一级里你将体会到彻底的精疲力竭，这一级你无法持久，就算持久了对你也没什么好处。

You should notreach level 10, for in this level, you will experience a total exhaustion.You should not go through exercise at such level, and even if you do try to maintain such intensity, it will not do you any good.

4.相对强度

Relative Intensity

（1）相对强度的定义

Definition

相对强度是指与个体能力相适应的负荷强度，常用个人的最大摄氧量、最大心率或心脏功能能力的百分数来表示。运动强度的确定必须依据个人的运动能力。能够达到改善心血管和呼吸功能的最低运动强度称为有效强度，最高强度可称为安全强度。只有达到了有效强度的运动，才能真正达到健身的目的，而超过安全强度的运动，则会危害身体的健康。

Relative intensity refers to the load intensity that corresponds to an individual's ability. It is often expressed as a percentage of an individual's MaximumVO2, MaximumHeart Rate, or Cardiac Functional Capacity. The intensity of exercise must be determined according to the individual's capability. The minimum intensity of exercise that can improve cardiovascular and respiratory function is called effective intensity, while the highest intensity is called safe intensity. Only to achieve the effective intensity of exercise, one can really achieve the purpose of exercising, and once the intensity surpass the level of safe intensity, such exercise can be harmful to our body.

（2）相对强度的测量内容及方法

相对运动强度指标	适宜运动强度范围（I）	测试方法
最大心率（MHR）	60%~90%	I*（220-年龄）或直接测定MHR
最大摄氧量（MaximumVO^2）	50%~85%	I*直接测定MaximumVO^{2}max

相对运动强度指标	适宜运动强度范围（I）	测试方法
心脏功能能力（MET）	50%~85%	I*（Maximum VO^2/3.5）
心率储备（HRR）	50%~85%	I*（MHR−安静HR）+安静HR
主观感觉量表（RPE）	12~16	

Measurement Content and Method of Relative Strength

Relative Intensity Index	Suitable Limitation	Method
MHR	60%~90%	I*（220−age）or measure MHR
Maximum VO^2	50%~85%	I*Maximum VO^2
MET	50%~85%	I*（Maximum VO^2/3.5）
HRR	50%~85%	I*（MHR−Rest HR）+Rest HR
RPE	12~16	

（二）肌肉力量和耐力的测量途径

Measurement of Muscle Strength and Endurance

1. 肌肉力量的测量

Measurement of Muscle Strength

（1）肌肉力量的定义

Definition

肌肉力量是指机体依靠肌肉收缩克服和对抗阻力来完成运动的能力。

Muscle strength refers to the ability of the body to overcome and counteract resistance through muscle contractions.

（2）肌肉力量的测量内容与方法

Contents and Methods of Measurement of Muscle Strength

肌肉力量的测量与评价一般包括等长肌力、等张肌力、等速肌力以及动力测量。

The measurement and evaluation of muscle strength generally include isotonic force, isometricforce, isokineticforce and dynamic measurement.

① 等长肌力测量

Isometric Measurement of Strength

等长肌力测量，是在肌肉收缩保持其长度不变时，将所能负担的最大负荷。测量指标主要包括握力、背力、臂力和腿部力量等，通常的测量手段主要有握力计、背力计等。等长肌力测量方法包括，握力等长测试，前臂及手部肌群的等长力量主要由握力的大小来反映，同时表达的是受试者前臂及手部肌肉的抓握能力；背力等长测试，背力测试主要体现人体背部伸肌群的等长力量，测量的也是背部肌群的最大力量；腿力等长测试，腿力测试作为下肢肌肉力量的反映，测试以伸膝力量为主，是股四头肌的最大等长收缩力量。

Isometric measurement of strength is measured by the maximum load that can be borne when the muscle remains its length during contraction. The measurement indexes mainly include grip strength, back strength, arm strength and leg strength, etc., and the usuallycan be measured through grip and back dynamograph, etc. The isometric muscle strength measurement methods include: Grip Strength Isometric Test, in which the isometric muscle strength of forearm and hand is mainly reflected by the size of grip strength, and it also expresses the grasping ability of forearm and hand muscles of subjects; Back Force Isometric Test, which mainly reflects the human back extensor group of equal length strengthand the maximum strength of back muscle group; Leg Force Isometric Test, which mainly focuses on knee extension strength as a reflection of lower limb muscle strength, referring to the maximum isometric contraction force of quadriceps.

② 等张肌力测量

Isotonic Measurement of Strength

等张肌力测量，是根据肌肉等张收缩时产生关节运动的特点，在被测肢体上施加可度量的重量作为阻力、肌肉收缩时所能带动的最大重量即为该肌肉的等张肌力。其测量方法包括最大等张肌力检测、肌耐力检测和肌肉功率检测。最大等张肌力检测可通过卧推、蹬腿、屈臂、负重蹲起等形式以1RM的表示方法进行检测；肌耐力检测，以70%1RM重量，重复练习，记录练习次数表示。也可采用俯卧撑、仰卧起坐、单杠引体向上等形式进行测量；肌肉功率检测可以借助立定跳远、纵跳摸高、小球掷远等方法测量。

Isotonic measurement of strength is based on the characteristics of joint movement during the isotonic contraction of muscles. A measurable weight applied to the measured limb as resistance as the maximum weight that can be driven by muscle contraction is the isotonic force of the muscle. The measurementmethods include maximum isotonic force test, muscle endurance test and muscle power test. Maximum isotonic strength can be measured by bench pressing, kicking, arm bending, squatting and other forms with 1RM representation. Muscle endurance was measured by repeated exercisesunder 70% 1RM weight, and the number of exercises will berecorded. It can also be measured in the forms of push-ups, sit-ups and horizontal bar pull-ups. The muscle power can be measured by means of standing long jump, vertical jump touch height, ball throwing distance and so on.

③等速肌力测量

Isokinetic Measurement of Strength

等速肌力测量，是在肢体进行等速运动时，测定肌肉的肌力等参数，来判断相关的肌肉、关节等的运动功能的方法。等速肌力测试包括，慢等速肌力测试、快等速肌力测试、等速离心肌力测试、等速向心肌力测试。测量等速肌肉力量一般使用等速肌肉测试训练仪。当肢体主动运动时，欲保持其速度不变，则肌力强时，杠杆的阻力大，从而，肌肉负荷大，肌张力高，力矩（肢体绕关节转动时，肢体的力量与用力点到关节垂直距离的乘积）输出增加；反之，当肌力弱时，杠杆的阻力随之减小，肌肉负荷亦降低，肌张力低，力矩输出减少。因此，当肢体被限制在不同的速度下进行等速运动时，测定力矩等参数，可判定肢体肌肉的功能状况。

Isokinetic measurement of strength is the determination of muscle strength and other parameters to judge the function of relevant muscles, joints, etc. The isokinetic muscle strength test includes slow isokinetic muscle strength test, fast isokinetic muscle strength test, isokinetic centrifugal muscle strength test, and isokinetic concentric muscle strength test. Isokinetic muscle strength is usually measured throughan isokinetic muscle test trainer. When the limb moves actively, to maintain the current speed, the resistance of the lever willincrease when the muscle strength is strong,thus, leading to more loads on the muscle and high musical tension, and the torque (the product of the limb's force and the vertical distance from the force point to the joint when the limb rotates around the joint) output will increase. On the contrary, when the muscle strength is weak, the resistance of the lever willreduce, leading to a reduction on the muscle load and low muscle tension.The torque output will also reduce. Therefore, while doing isokinetic activities at different speed level, the function of the limb muscles can be determined by measuring parameters such as torque.

④ 动力测试

Dynamic Test

动力性力量测试中受试者可以用爆发用力的形式对抗身体、肢体或是外加质量惯性，测试中阻力或阻抗质量保持不变，对测试速度与加速度没有限制，所以可以较为准确地反映人体负重时肌肉的收缩与放松过程。但是，动力性肌肉力量要比静力性力量更加难以描述和控制。而动态功率的变化可量化特定肌群短时间内的快速做功能力，以及肌肉长时间持续工作时的耐久力。肌肉输出功率为扭矩与角速度的乘积，因此力量—速度关系曲线能反映出肌肉功率输出能力的机能特征。在一系列预负荷阻力设置的测试中，预负荷（阻力矩值）与测试系统的角速度呈线性关系，且肌肉向心收缩过程中力量与角速度成反比关系，收缩速度的增加会伴随着肌肉力量的降低。

In dynamic test, test subjects will use power against the body, and limbs or external mass inertia. During the test, resistance or impedance mass will remainunchanged. There is no limit onspeed and acceleration. Therefore, such testcan reflect the process of muscle contraction and relaxation when body carries weight. However, dynamic muscle force is more difficult to describe and control than static force. Dynamic power quantifies the ability of a particular muscle group to react over a short period of time, as well as themuscle enduranceover a long period of time. The muscle output power is the product of torque and angular velocity.So, the force-velocity curve can reflect the functional characteristics of muscle power output ability. In a series of tests with preload resistance setting, the preload (resistance moment value)is linearly related to the angular velocity of the test system, and the force is inversely proportional to the angular velocity during the centroid contraction of the muscle, and the increase of contraction speed is accompanied by the decrease of muscle strength.

（3）肌肉力量测试的注意事项及影响因素
Precautions and Influencing Factors in Muscle Strength Test

测试需要针对特定肌群进行测试，肌肉收缩类型、收缩速度、测试设备、关节活动范围、动作熟练程度等因素都会影响测试结果。

Specific muscle groups need to be tested. Factors such as type of muscle contraction, speed of contraction, test equipment, range of joint motion, and motor proficiency can affect the results of the test.

2. 肌肉耐力的测量
Measurement of Muscular Endurance

（1）肌肉耐力的定义
Definition

肌肉耐力是指人体长时间进行持续肌肉工作的能力，即对抗疲劳的能力。

Muscle endurance refers to the body's ability to perform sustained muscle work over a long period of time, i.e. the ability to resist fatigue.

（2）肌肉耐力的测量内容与方法
Measurement Content and Method of Muscle Endurance

肌肉耐力的测量与评价一般包括等长肌肉耐力、等张肌肉耐力以及等速肌肉耐力。测量综合阻力、时间、重复次数3个指标。

The measurement and evaluation of muscle endurance generally include isometric muscle endurance, isotonic muscle endurance and isokineticmuscle endurance. The comprehensive resistance, time and repetition times aremeasured.

① 等长肌肉耐力

Isometric Muscle Endurance

等长收缩是肌肉静力性工作的基础，在人体运动中对运动环节固定、支持和保持身体某种姿势起重要作用。等长肌肉耐力一般是以一定负荷所能坚持的时间长短来表示，如悬垂、倒立、平衡等各种姿势的保持时间。

Isometric contraction is the basis of static muscle work. It plays an important role in fixing, supporting and maintaining a certain posture of the body in the movement of human body. Isometric muscle endurance detection is generally indicated through the duration of a certain postureunder certain load, such as the holding time of various postures such as hanging, handstand and balance.

② 等张肌肉耐力

Isotonic Muscle Endurance

等张肌肉耐力的检测一般以1RM负荷重量的百分比（通常70%）为标准，然后让受试者重复完成规定的练习，记录练习次数，用以表示等张肌肉耐力水平。也可以采用常用的俯卧撑、仰卧起坐、单杠引体向上等练习次数，了解不同部位肌群活动的等张肌肉耐力水平。

The test of isotonic muscle endurance is generally based on the percentage of 1RM load weight(usually 70%). The subjects are asked to repeat a series ofprescribed exercises with the number of such exercise repeated recorded to indicate isotonic muscle endurance. You can also use push-ups, sit-ups, horizontal bar pull-ups, etc. to learnthe subjects' isotonic muscle endurance level of different parts of muscle group.

③等速肌肉耐力

Isokinetic Muscle Endurance

等速肌肉耐力的测量常用的方法有两种，耐力比测定，如以每秒180°关节运动角度连续做最大收缩25次，计其末5次（或10次）与首5次（或10次）做功量之比，称耐力比；50%衰减实验，以每秒180°或240°的速度连续做最大收缩，直到有2-5次不能达到最初5次运动平均峰力矩的50%时为止，以完成的运动次数作为肌肉耐力评价的参数。

There are two kinds of methods which arecommonly used during the isokinetic muscle endurance measurement. Endurance ratio measurement When doing such as a 180° joint motion angle per second with continuous maximum contraction for 25 times, count the last 5 times (or 10 times)and the first 5 times (or 10 times)work ratio, and such ratio can be used to indicateendurance ratio. 50% attenuation test A continuous maximum contraction is performed at a speed of 180° or 240° per second during the test until the subject has failed to reach 50% of the average peak torque of the first 5 movements for 2-5 times. The number of completed movements is taken as the parameter for the evaluation ofmuscle endurance.

④其他测量方面

Other Measurements

其他测量方面，传统测量方法中用可重复12RM的负荷测试耐力、通过给定频率，重复对抗阻力动作的次数以测量评定肌肉耐力水平。

In terms of other measurements, the traditional measurement method uses repeated 12-RM load to test endurance, and the number of repeated anti-resistance movements to measure and assess the level of muscle endurance through a given frequency.

思考

Questions

1. 健康测量的常用操作技术包括哪些？请简要回答。

What are the common operation techniques for health measurement? Please answer briefly.

2. 高尿酸血症高危人群建议多久进行一次筛查？

How often are screening recommended for people at high risk for hyperuricemia?

3. 列举一些健康测量的常用操作，并且说明其在健康促进中的作用。

List some common operations of health measurement and explain its role in health promotion.

第五章　健康教育与健康促进
CHAPTER FIVE HEALTH EDUCATION AND HEALTH PROMOTION

健康促进与健康教育是全民素质教育的重要内容，是解决社会主要公共卫生问题的重要手段，也是"21世纪人人享有卫生保健"目标的战略性策略。通过健康促进与健康教育，营造有益于健康的环境，提高广大人民群众的健康意识和自我保健能力，对于减少和消除健康危险因素，预防和控制重大疾病及突发公共卫生事件，保护和增进人民健康，提高人口健康素质具有重要的意义。

Health education and health promotion are important content in public liberal education as well as an important means to solve major public health issues in society, and are alsoa strategy for reaching the goal of "Health Care for All in the 21st Century". Through health education and health promotion, the goal is to create a healthy environment, and to improve people's health consciousness and self-care ability. It is of great impartance in health risk factors reduction and elimination, major diseases and public health emergencies prevention, and public health improvement.

第一节　健康行为
Section One Health Behaviour

一、健康行为的概念

Concept on Health Behavio

广义的健康行为是指一切与健康或疾病有关的行为，其中可分为直接或者间接影响健康的个体行为和群体行为。狭义的健康行为是指个体在工作生活中采取的行为,这种行为将会对个体的生理或心理健康产生直接或间接的影响。

依据1978年WHO阿拉木图宣言中的健康概念,健康应包含四个层次:生理健康、心理健康、道德健康、社会适应健康。健康行为亦应基于上述四方面界定。

Health behavior refers to all behaviors related to health or disease, which can be divided into individual behavior and group behavior that directly or indirectly affect health. Health behaviors can also be explained in a narrower sense as the behaviors taken by individuals in their work and life, that have direct or indirect impact on his or her physical or mental health.

According to the concept of health in the 1978 Declaration of Alma-Ata, health should have four aspects, including physical health, mental health, moral health and health of society adaptability. Health behavior should also be defined on the basis of the above four aspects.

二、健康行为分析的注意事项

Precautions for Health Behavior Analysis

从行为医学角度,分析健康行为应考虑:

From the perspective of behavioral medicine, we should consider the following factors when analyzing health behaviors:

(一)健康行为应包括人的身、心、社会方面均健康时的外在表现

Health Behavior Should Include the One's External Performance of Physical, Mental and Social Health

躯体健康的人,行为反应灵敏,活动精力充沛,心理健康的人情绪活动有较强的自我控制力,思维言语符合理性,精神面貌正常,而社会健康的人其行为符合社会规范。

Physically healthy people should be fast-reacting and energetic. Mentally healthy people should have strong self-control in emotion, the ability for rational thinking and speaking, and a positive attitude towards life.

（二）健康行为要求不影响自己、他人乃至整个社会的健康

Health Behavior Requires One to HaveNoNegative Impact on the Health of Oneself, Others and the Society

一个基本符合身、心健康的人，其诸方面的行为表现都应在常态水平及正向方向上，符合伦理道德规范，不能给他人或社会带来不良影响。

A physically and mentally healthy person should behavior morally and positively, causing no negative impacts on others or the society.

（三）能及时准确感受外界条件的改变，正确调整自己的行为

One Should Be Able to Perceivethe Change of External Conditions Timely and Accurately, and Adjust Accordingly

人处于不断变化的自然环境与社会环境，不同的情况下要以相应的行为对外界条件发生反应。

People are in anever-changing environment, and thus, theyhave to react to external conditions with corresponding behaviors.

三、健康行为的特征

Characteristics of Health Behaviour

（一）有利性

Advantage

有利性是指行为表现能产生积极的效果，对自身、他人、环境能够带来积极的影响。

Advantage refers to the positive effect ofbehaviorson oneself, others and the environment.

（二）规律性

Regularity

规律性行为指生活有节奏，处于平衡态，包括起居有常、饮食有节等行为。

Regularity refers to a habitual life in balance, including regular daily life.

（三）合理性

Rationality

合理性指行为表现可被自己、他人和社会所理解和接受。

Rationality means that one's behavior can be understood and accepted by oneself, others and society.

（四）方向准确性

Directional Accuracy

行为方向准确性指行为强度一般在正常水平上，包括语言表达行为、情绪行为、工作行为等。

The directional accuracy of behaviors means that the intensity of behaviors is generally in the normal level, including language expression, emotion, work, etc.

（五）同一性

Identity

同一性表现在外在行为与内在思维动机协调一致，并且与所处的环境条件无冲突。

Identity is embodied in the harmony between external behavior and internal thinking motivation with no conflict against the environmental conditions.

（六）整体和谐性

Integral Harmony

行为整体和谐性指个人行为具有的固有特征，与他人或环境发生冲突时，表现出容忍和适应。

The overall harmony of behavior is the inherent characteristics of one's personal behaviors. When people conflict with others and the environment, they should show tolerance and adaptation.

四、健康行为的影响因素

Influential Factors on Health Behaviour

任何健康行为都受倾向因素、促成因素以及强化因素三大因素的影响，这为我们平时的健康行为干预提供了方向。在健康教育工作中必须认真分析三类因素的影响，在发扬正向因素积极作用的同时，把干预重点放到负向影响上。

Any health behavior can be affected by three major factors: tendency factor, contributing factor and reinforcing factor.These three factors provide a direction for health behavior intervention. In the work of health education, the influence of these three factors must be carefully analyzed, and any intervention should focus on eliminating the negative influence on healthandreinforcing positive factors.

（一）倾向因素

Tendency Factors

倾向因素指健康的愿望、信念、知识和态度等，主要是指主观因素。

Tendency factors refer to the desire, belief, knowledge and attitude towards health, mainly refers to subjective factors.

（二）促成因素

Contributing Factors

促成因素指使健康愿望得以实现的因素，如生活环境、物质条件、拥有的健康相关技能等，主要是指相关的客观条件。

Contributing factors refer to the factors that enable the realization of desires on health,such as living environment, material conditions, health related skills, etc., mainly refer to objective conditions.

（三）强化因素

Intensified Factors

强化因素指家人或周围朋友对健康行为实施奖励或惩罚措施，以便使该行为得到支持或反对的因素，主要是指第三方因素。

Reinforcingfactors refer to the rewards and punishments from family members or friends in order to reinforce or eliminate certain behaviors, mainly refers to the third party factors.

第二节 健康教育
Section Two Health Education

一、健康教育的概念
Concept on Health Education

健康教育是通过信息传播和行为干预,帮助个体或群体掌握卫生保健知识,树立健康观念,自愿采纳有利于健康行为和生活方式的教育活动过程,消除或减轻影响健康的危险因素,预防疾病、促进健康和提高生活质量。健康教育的内容主要集中于一般性健康教育、特殊性健康教育和卫生管理法规教育。健康教育是一种以健康为中心的全民教育,通过使社会人群参与,改变其认知态度和价值观念,从而使其自觉采取有益于健康的行为和生活方式。

Health education refers to education process designed to help individuals or groups to master health care knowledge, establish health concepts, voluntarily adopt healthy behavior and lifestyle. It is to eliminate or reduce risk factors affecting health, prevent diseases, promote health and improve the quality of life. The content of health education mainly focuses on general health education, special health education and health management regulation education. Health education is a kind of health-centered public education. Through the participation of social groups, the public will change their cognition and values, eventually adopting healthy behavior and lifestyle consciously.

二、健康教育的目的
Health Education Objectives

健康教育目的是通过健康教育活动的过程,达到改善、维护和促进个体和社会的健康状况和文明建设的程度;增进人们的健康,使个人和群体为实现健康目标而努力;提高或维护健康,增强自我保健力;预防非正常死亡、疾病和残疾的发生。主要包括增进个体和群体对健康的认识，鼓励采取和维持健康的生活方式，有效利用卫生保健资源，改善生活环境和人际关系和增强自我保健意识和能力。

The purpose of health education is to improve, maintain and promote individual and social health as well ascivilization construction through the process of health education and health promotion activities. Through health education, the public health can be improved with every individual and social group working towards the goal of health. The ability of self-care can be enhanced. It can also prevent individual's unnatural death, diseases and disabilities.Health educationincludes promoting health awareness of individuals and groups, encouraging the adoption and maintenance of healthy lifestyles, effective use of health-care resources, improving living conditions andinterpersonal relationships, and enhancing self-awareness and capacity for health care.

三、健康教育的内容

Content of Health Education

健康教育的内容有以下三类，即一般性健康教育，是为了帮助了解个人和人群健康的基本知识；特殊性健康教育，即针对社区特殊人群常见的健康问题进行教育；卫生管理法规教育，帮助人们了解法规，提高责任心和自觉性。

The main content of health education has the following three categories. General health education: to master the basic knowledge of individual and population health. Special health education: to educate special people in the community on the common health problems. Education on health regulations: to understand the laws and regulations, and to improve the sense of responsibility and consciousness.

四、健康教育的方法

Methods of Health Education

要根据不同年龄、性别、职业、文化程度、对保健知识的求知欲等采取不同的健康教育方法。健康教育的方法很多，主要包括以下几种：

Different methods of health education should be adopted according to different age, sex, occupation, educational level and desire for knowledge of health care. Methods of health education can be divided into the followings:

（一）语言健康教育法

Language Health Education

语言健康教育法是通过面对面的口头语言进行直接教育的方法。主要通过交谈、小组讨论、健康咨询、专题讲座等形式开展。

The language health education is a method of face-to-face education, which is mainly conducted through conversation, group discussion, healthconsultation, special lectures, etc.

（二）文字健康教育法

Text Health Education

文字健康教育法是以文字或图片为工具，将健康知识文字印刷成报纸、图画、宣传卡片或宣传手册等，通过简明、形象、生动的文字描述使人们易于接受和掌握，从而达到健康教育目的的一种方法。

The text health education is a method that takes the text or the picture as the tool for health education. Health knowledge is printed as newspaper, pictures, memory cards or brochures, etc. Through brief and vivid word descriptions, people can easily accept relevant health knowledge, achieving the purpose of health education.

（三）形象化教育法

Visualization Education

形象化教育法是以各种形式的艺术造型直接刺激人的视觉器官，以及使用生动的文字说明或口头解释，通过人的视觉及听觉而作用于人的大脑的教育方法，如音频材料、演示等。

Visualization education method relies on the direct effect of visual art on humans. Through visualized images and vivid word or oral explanation, one can access relevant health knowledge through sight and hearing. Such method can be conducted through audio teaching materials, live demonstration, etc.

除了以上三种教育方法外，网络教育和案例学习也是实现健康教育目的的有效手段。健康教育可采取单一方式进行，也可采取多种方式进行，灵活运用各种方法以达到既能使受教育者易于接受，又能产生良好效果的预期目的。

In addition to these three methods, online education and case study are also effective methods to achieve the purpose of health education. Health education can be carried out through single methods or combined styles. Flexibly applying multiple teaching methods can allow learners an easier access to health knowledge and thus achieves the teaching purposes.

五、健康教育的原则

Principles of Health Education

健康教育是一种特殊的教育，教育者通过有目的、有组织、有计划的系统活动，把健康知识传播给公众，唤起公众的健康意识，从而使人们树立对自己及社会的责任感，投入到卫生保健活动中来。在实施健康教育时应遵循以下几个原则：

Health education is a special kind of education. Educators aim to spread health knowledge to public and arouse public health awareness through purpose-oriented, organized and planned systematic activities, so as to help the public establish a sense of responsibility and devote themselves into health-care activities. The following principles should be followed in the implementation of health education:

（一）科学实用

Principle of Being Scientific and Practical

科学实用原则是指健康教育所传播的知识要能够有效帮助受教育者树立健康意识，掌握了解生活中常见疾病的基本技能。

The principle of being scientific and practical refers to that the health knowledge should be effective to establish individual's health awareness with the mastery of the basic understandings on common diseases.

（二）因材施教
Principle of Adapted Teaching Methods

因材施教原则是指开展健康教育必须按照各类人群不同的学习需求和学习起点，设计不同的教育方式和内容。

The principle of adapted teaching methods means that different teachingmethods and contents must be designed according to different learners and their specific conditions.

（三）寓教于乐
Principle of Education for Fun

寓教于乐原则是指健康教育应该结合在行动、情景、乐趣之中，应该要以健康行为实践为中心，通过实践来激发受教育者的学习热情。

Theprinciple of education for fun means that health education should be conducted throughpractice andactual scenes, with fun, and should focus on the practice of health behaviors to stimulate the enthusiasm of learners through practice.

（四）启发诱导
Principle of Inspiration and Induction

启发诱导原则是指在进行健康教育过程中，要以受教育者为主体，调动他们的学习主动性，引导他们独立思考，积极探索，自觉地掌握健康知识，提高解决健康问题的能力。

The principle of inspiration and induction refers that in the process of health education, learners should be in the leading position, and thus, teachers should inspire their learning initiative, guide them to think independently and to actively explore issues, help them consciously master health knowledge and improve the ability to solve health problems.

（五）循序渐进
Principle of Gradual Learning

循序渐进原则是指健康教育要按照逻辑系统和受教育者认识发展的顺序进行，使其逐渐系统地掌握基础知识和基本技能。

The principle of gradual learning means that health education should be carried out in accordance with the logic and the cognition development of learners. To do so, learners can gradually and systematically master the basic knowledge and basic skills.

（六）社区参与

Principle of Community Participation

社区参与原则是指要鼓励教育对象积极参与社区健康教育教学活动，目的是改变教育对象的不健康的生活行为及方式。

The principle of community participation refers to encouraging people to actively participate in community health education and teaching activities with the purpose of changing their unhealthy lifestyles.

（七）程序性

Principle of Procedure

程序性原则是指把健康教育基础知识分成一系列连续模块进行学习，安排由浅入深，由简到繁，逐一掌握健康知识技能。

The principle of procedure means that the basic health knowledge should be divided into a series of continuous learning modules, from shallow to deep, from simple to complex, allowing learners to master health knowledge and relevant skills step by step.

六、健康教育的相关理论模式

Relevant Theoretical Models of Health Education

（一）知—信—行模式（KABP或HAP模式）

Knowledge-Attitude-Practice Model（KABP or HAP Model）

知—信—行模式也称为认知行为目标模式（Knowledge，Attitude，Belief，Practice，简称KABP或KAP）是美国Barbara A. Carper教授于1978年提出的。知—信—行模式是改变人类健康相关行为的模式之一，它将人类行为的改变分为获取知识、产生信念及形成行为3个连续过程。"知"是知识、信息，"信"是正确的信念和积极的态度，"行"是产生促进健康的行为。

知—信—行模式认为知识是基础，信念是动力，行为的产生和改变是目标。其基本理念是人们通过学习，获得相关的健康知识和技能，逐步形成健康的信念和态度，从而促成健康行为的产生。

The Knowledge-Attitude-Practice Model (KAP), also known as the Cognitive Behavioral Model (Knowledge, Attitude, Belief, Practice, or KAP for short), was proposed by American Professor Barbara A. Carper in 1978. The Knowledge-Attitude-Practice Model is one of the models that changed human health-related behaviors. It divides the changes of human behavior into three continuous processes: knowledge acquisition, belief generation and behavior formation. K is the knowledge as well as information. A is the right faith and positive attitude. P is the generation of health-promoting behavior. The Knowledge-Attitude-Practice Model holds that knowledge is the foundation while belief is the motivation, and the generation and change of behaviors is the goal. The basic idea is that people acquire relevant health knowledge and skills through learning, and gradually form healthy beliefs and attitudes. Eventually, based on these beliefs, one can change his or her health behavior.

（二）健康信念模式（HBM模式）

Health Belief Model (HBM Model)

健康信念模式（HBM模式）是第一个解释和预测健康行为的理论，由三位社会心理学家霍克鲍姆、罗森斯托克和凯格尔在1952年提出。关注人对健康的态度和信念，重视影响信念的内外因素。健康信念模式认为健康信念是人们接受劝导、改变不良行为，采纳健康促进行为的基础和关键。它的特点在于应用心理学方法解释健康相关行为、遵照认知理论、强调人体主观心理过程对行为的主导作用。健康信念模式主要内容包括：感知到疾病的易感性；感知到疾病的严重性；感知到健康行为的效益；感知到健康行为的障碍；感知到自我效能；影响因素，指来自社会人口学、社会心理学的影响；提示因素，指诱发健康行为发生的各类因素，包括媒体宣传、劝告、医务人员提醒等。

The Health Belief Model (HBM Model) is the first theory to explain and predict health behaviors. It was proposed by three social psychologists,

Hochbaum, Rosenstock and Kegels, in 1952. This model pays attention to people's attitudes and beliefs on health, and focuses on the internal and external factors that affect beliefs on health. Health belief model holds that health belief is the key for people to accept persuasion, to change bad behavior and to adopt health promotion behavior. It is characterized by applying psychological methods to explain health-related behaviors, complying with cognitive theories, and emphasizing the leading role of human subjective psychological processes. The main contents of health belief model include: perception of disease susceptibility; perceiving the severity of the disease; perceived benefits of healthy behaviors; perceived barriers to healthy behavior; perceived self-efficacy; influencing factors, which refers to the influences from social demography and social psychology; cue factors, which are all kinds of factors that induce healthy behavior, such as media publicity, advice, medical personnel remind, etc.

（三）格林模式（PRECEDE-PROCEED模式）

Precede-Proceed Model

格林（Precede-Proceed）模式，由美国著名的健康教育学家劳伦斯·格林（Lawrence W. Green）提出。格林模式具有两个特点：一是其为从结果入手的程序，即用演绎的方法进行推理思考——从最终的结果追溯到最初的起因，先问"为什么"，再问"如何去进行"，避免以主观猜测代替一系列的需求诊断。二是考虑了影响健康的多重因素，显示出一切个人和群体行为与环境变革的努力，必须是多元的，因此健康教育与健康促进计划的设计也应该是多层面的。格林模式主要包含两个阶段：一是PRECEDE阶段，重点在于评估诊断行为原因。在教育诊断和评估中应用倾向因素、促进因素及强化因素。二是PROCEED阶段，关注实施过程和评价。在执行教育/环境干预中应用政策、法规和组织手段。格林模式分为以下七个步骤：社会诊断；流行病学诊断；行为和环境诊断；教育和组织诊断；管理和政策诊断；实施教育计划；评价阶段。

Precede-Proceed Model was raised by the famous American health educator Lawrence W. Green. Precede-Proceed Model has two characteristics. One is that it is a procedure that starts with the result. That is to reason with deductive method, tracing back to the original cause from the final result, asking "why" first, and then "how to proceed", to avoid replacing a series of needs diagnosis with subjective guess. The second is to consider the multiple factors affecting health, showing that all individual and group behaviors and environmental changing efforts must be multi-faceted. Therefore, the design of health education and health promotion programs should also be multi-faceted. Precede-Proceed Model consists of two stages. First is the PRECEDE stage, which emphasizes on assessing the causes of diagnostic behavior. The tendency factors, the promotion factors and the intensified factors are applied in the education diagnosis and assessment. The second is PROCEED stage, which focus on implementation process and evaluation, applying policies, regulations and organizational tools in the implementation of educational/environmental interventions. Precede-Proceed Model is divided into seven steps, including social diagnosis, epidemiological diagnosis, behavioral and environmental diagnosis, education and organizational diagnosis, management and policy diagnosis, education plan and evaluation stage.

其中教育与组织诊断包括以下三个步骤：第一步分析影响因素；第二步确定优先项目顺序；第三步制定干预重点。

Educational and organizational diagnosis includes the following three steps: influencing factors analysis, determining the order of priorities, formulating the focus of intervention.

第三节　健康促进
Section Three Health Promotion

一、健康促进的概念
Concept of Health Promotion

健康促进是指一切能促使行为和生活条件向有益于健康改变的教育和生

态支持的综合体。健康促进可以理解为是健康教育与环境因素共同作用的结果，也可以理解为是健康教育和行政手段共同作用的结果。健康促进是指个人与家庭、社区和国家一起采取措施鼓励健康的行为，增强人们改进和处理自身健康问题的能力。

According to Lawrence Green, health promotion is a complex of education and ecological supports that promotes behavior and living conditions to health-friendly changes. Health promotion can be interpreted as the result of health education and environmental factors as well as the administrative means. Health promotion means that individuals, together with families, communities and society, take measures to encourage health behavior and enhance people's ability to improve and deal with their own health problems.

二、健康促进的任务

Health Promotion Tasks

健康促进在推进健康上的主要任务有：

From the perspective of promoting health construction, the main tasks in health promotion are as follows:

（一）制定健康公共政策

Formulating Public Policies for Health

制定健康公共政策是指必须将促进健康的理念融入公共政策制定实施的全过程。坚持以人的健康为中心，针对主要健康问题和健康需求，制定有利于健康的公共政策，将健康相关内容纳入各项建设和管理之中。

The formulation of public policy on health means that the concept of health promotion must be integrated into the whole process of the formulation and implementation of public policy. Adhere to people's health as the center according to the main health problems and health needs, and establish public policies conducive to health, and bring health-related content into the construction and management of all.

（二）创造支持性环境
Creating a Supportive Environment

创造支持性环境是指为达到健康目的，提供便利或帮助，创造有利的外部因素，主要包括改善物质条件、社会环境、政治环境等。

Creating a supportive environment can provide the public convenience to achieve the goal of health with favorable external factors, mainly including improving the material conditions, social environment and political environment.

（三）强化社区行动
Intensifying Community Actions

强化社区行动是指调动社区居民带头人，以社区为单位开展活动，发掘社区资源，进行社区教育，提供社区居民活动参与度。

Intensifying community action refers to encouraging the community leaders to carry out activities with the participation of the community members, exploring community resources, and conducting community education.

（四）发展个人技能
Developing Personal Skills

发展个人技能主要是指普及健康相关知识，提高个人健康意识和个人生活技能，使人具备解决日常生活中各种健康需求的技能。

Developing personal skills mainly refers to the popularization of health-related knowledge as well as the improvement of personal health awareness and personal life skills so that the public may have the skills to solve daily health needs.

（五）调整卫生服务方向
Adjusting the Direction of Health Services

调整卫生服务方向是指卫生机构需要根据居民新的健康需求为导向，使用各种卫生资源向居民提供医疗、预防、保健、康复服务。

Adjusting the direction of health services means that health institutions need to use various health resources to provide residents with medical treatment, disease prevention, health care and rehabilitation services based on the new health needs of residents.

三、健康促进的策略

Strategies for Health Promotion

健康促进是一个增强人们控制影响健康的因素，改善自身健康的能力的过程，健康促进策略包括基本策略和核心策略。

Health promotion is a process to enhance people's ability to control factors affecting their health and improve their own health. Health promotion strategies include basic strategies and core strategies.

（一）基本策略

Basic Strategies

健康促进的基本策略包含倡导、赋权及协调三种方式。倡导指一种有组织的个体及社会的联合行动；赋权指实现健康人权的平等；协调指促进各部门的利益协调一致。

The basic strategy of health promotion includes three ways: advocacy, empowerment and coordination. Advocacy refers to an organized collective action from both individuals and the society. Empowerment refers to the realization of the equal rights to health. Coordination means to reach an consensus on the interests amorg various departments.

（二）核心策略

Core Strategies

健康促进的核心策略主要是社会动员。即领导层的动员、专业部门和人员参与的动员、非政府组织的动员以及社区、家庭与个人参与的动员。

The core strategy of health promotion is mainly social motivation, which includes motivation on leadership, motivation on professional departments and personnel, motivation on non-governmental organizations and motivation on community, family as well asindividual participation.

第四节 健康传播
Section Four Health Transmission

一、健康传播的概念
Concept of Health Communication

健康传播是以"人人健康"为出发点，运用各种传播媒介渠道和方法，为维护和促进人类健康的目的而制作、传递、分散、分享健康信息的过程。健康传播是健康教育和健康促进的重要手段与策略。

Health communication is a process of making, transmitting, dispersing and sharing health information for the purpose of maintaining and promoting public through various media channels. Health communication is an important means and strategy for health education and health promotion.

二、健康传播的目的
Purpose of Health Communication

健康传播的目标为传得快、传即通、传有效。按可达到的难度层次由低到高分为4个层次：知晓信息，是最低层次的传播效果；信念认同，是价值观念的基础；态度向有利于健康转变，这是行为的先导；采纳健康的行为和生活方式，这是最高层次传播效果。

The goal of health communication is to spread the health information quickly, smoothly and effectively. It can be divided into four levels from low difficulty to high. Knowing the information is the lowest level of communication effect. Belief identity is the basis of values. A change in attitude to what is good for health is the precursor to action. Adopting healthy behaviors and lifestyles is the highest level of communication effect.

三、健康传播的影响因素

Factors Affecting Health Transmission

健康传播的影响因素包含五个方面，分别为：

The influencing factors of health transmission include five aspects.

（一）健康传播者方面

Communicators

健康传播者自身业务素质要高，要发挥好健康信息的把关人作用，所以选择合适的传播者显得尤为重要。

Health communicators should have highly professional and play a good role as a gatekeeper of health information. Therefore, it is particularly important to choose the right communicators.

（二）健康信息方面

Health Information

首先要保证信息内容具有针对性、科学性和指导性。其次，使用符号要准确、通用、适合受传者与媒介采用。同时信息表达形式的设计应符合传播目的和受传者需求。注意符号和信息的抽象度，要与目标人群的知识结构和理解能力相对应。

First of all, we must ensure that health information is targeted, scientific and instructive. Secondly, the choices on words for health information should be accurate, understandable and appropriate. At the same time, the design of information expression should conform to the purpose of communication and the needs of receivers. Attention should be paid to the abstraction of symbols, ensuring that health information delivered should be corresponded to the knowledge structure and understanding ability of the target population.

（三）媒介渠道方面

Media Channels

要注意媒介渠道的选择，充分考虑目标人群的适应性。采取多媒介渠道的组合策略，多层次多渠道地开发利用媒体。

Attention should be paid to the selection of media channels. The adaptability of the target population should be fully considered. We can adopt the combination of multiple media channels as the spreading strategy.

（四）受传者方面

Receivers

健康传播的受众是社会人群，他们有着不同的健康需求和信息需求。了解受传者在知晓、劝服、采纳、加强不同阶段的心理因素，把握受传者在接收信息传播过程中的共同心理特征，熟悉受传者的社会经济文化特征，掌握受传者的健康状况。根据受众的生理与心理特点制定相应的传播策略。

The receivers of health communication are social groups who have different health needs and information needs. We should understand the different psychological levels of the receivers in knowing, persuading, adopting and strengthening stages; the common psychological characteristics of the receivers should be grasped in the process of receiving information dissemination. Communicators should be familiar with the social, economic and cultural characteristics of the receivers, and grasp the health status of the receivers. Corresponding communication strategies according to the physiological and psychological characteristics of the receivers should be formulated.

（五）环境方面

Environment

传播活动赖以生存的自然环境和社会环境是传播过程中不可忽略的要素之一。自然环境通常指传播活动地点、场所、距离和环境布置等，社会环境主要指社会经济状况、文化习俗、政策法规等。

The natural and social environment which communication activities depend on is one of the elements that cannot be ignored in the process of communication. The natural environment usually refers to the location, place, distance and environmental layout of communication activities, while the social environment mainly refers to the social and economic conditions, cultural customs, policies and regulations, etc.

第五节 社区健康教育
Section Five Community Health Education

一、社区健康教育的概念与步骤
Concept and Steps of Community Health Education

社区健康教育是以社区为基本单位，以社区人群为教育对象，以促进居民健康为目标，有计划、有组织、有评价的教育活动。社区健康教育程序包括社区健康教育评估、社区健康教育诊断/问题、社区健康教育计划、社区健康教育实施、社区健康教育评价五个步骤。

Community health education is a planned, organized and evaluated educational activity within a community. With community groups as the targets of education, the goal is to promote the residents' health. The program of community health education includes five steps: community health education evaluation, community health education diagnosis, community health education planning, community health education implementation, community health education scoring.

二、社区健康教育评估的内容
Contents of Community Health Education Evaluation

社区健康教育评估内容包括以下四个方面：教育对象一般资料评估，如生活方式、学习能力、对健康认知与学习态度；教育环境评估，包括生活、学习和社会环境；健康服务状况评估，如健康医疗设施、健康服务条件；教育者评估，教育者能力、水平、经验。

The contents of community health education assessment include the following four aspects: the general information assessment of the education objects, such as lifestyle, learning ability, health cognition and learning attitude; assessment on the educational environment, including the living, learning and social environment; assessment onthe status of health services, such as health facilities, health conditions; assessment on educators, including their teaching ability and teaching experience.

三、社区健康问题的确定
Identification of Community Health Issues

社区健康问题的确定是社区健康教育计划与实施的前提。确定问题首先要提出问题、指出与健康相关行为的影响因素，找出社区健康教育问题根源后再根据该问题对人群健康威胁的严重性、危险因素的可干预程度、成本效益分析三个维度来确定优先项目。

The determination of community health issues is the premise of community health education plan and implementation. To determine the issues, first of all, we should put forward the problem and point out the influencing factors on health-related behaviors. Then, after finding out the cause of the community health education problem, we should determine the priority according to the seriousness of the threat to the public health, the possibility on interfering risk factors and the cost-benefit analysis.

四、社区健康教育的计划
Community Health Education Programs

开展社区健康教育工作，必须进行科学的设计，以明确目标，合理科学地安排工作程序，做到有的放矢，有计划、有步骤、有效地进行健康教育。这是达到健康教育目的的关键环节。社区健康教育计划包括制定健康教育目标、社区健康教育内容和预期结局、社区健康教育的活动时间、场所、对象和人数以及评价指标和标准。

To carry out the work of community health education, the project first should be designed scientifically with clear educational targets. Based on these targets, the working procedure should be arranged reasonably and scientifically, carrying out the health education effectively in a planned, orderly and effective way. This is the key to achieve the purpose of health education. The planning on community health education includes setting the goal of community health education, determining the teaching content and expected results, deciding the time, place, objects and number of community health education activities, as well as the determination on evaluation index and standards.

五、社区健康教育实施的前提与步骤

Premise and Steps of Implementing Community Health Education

（一）实施前提

Implementation Premise

社区健康教育的实施是在领导与社区相关工作人员共同组织下进行的，在实施工作开始之前，首先应完成实施工作时间表的制定。实施工作时间表是整个执行计划的核心，也是实现目标管理的体现，时间表也是一个对照表，可以用来对照检查各项工作的进展速度和完成数量。其次要做好培训课程及培训人员的安排工作。除此之外，充裕的物资准备也是保障顺利实施的前提条件。

The implementation of community health education is carried out under the joint organization of leaders and community related staff. Before the start of the implementation work, the implementation work schedule should be completed first. The implementation of the work schedule is the core of the entire implementation plan, and also the realization of management of objectives. The schedule is also a check table, which can be used to check the progress of the speed of work and the number of completion. Secondly, the arrangement of training courses and training personnel should be done well. In addition, adequate material preparation is also a prerequisite for the smooth implementation of the guarantee.

（二）实施步骤

Implementation Steps

社区健康教育实施具体实施步骤包括：开发领导层；提供良好的环境；鼓励教育对象积极参与；认真组织好教学的内容和材料准备；合理安排教学内容，遵循循序渐进的原则；严格控制质量，重视健康教育信息的反馈。

The specific implementation steps of community health education include: developing the leadership, providing a good environment, ensuring the active participation of educational objects, organizing the teaching content and material preparation carefully, arranging teaching content reasonably, following the principle of step by step, strictly controlling the quality and attaching importance to the feedback of health education information.

六、社区健康教育评价

Evaluation of Community Health Education

（一）社区健康教育评价的概念

Concept of Community Health Education Evaluation

健康教育评价是一个系统地收集、分析、展示资料的过程，它将贯穿于健康教育过程的始终。社区健康教育评价不仅能使我们了解健康教育项目的效果，还能全面监测、控制、保障社区健康教育计划的实施和实施质量，从而成为取得预期效果的关键措施。

Health education evaluation is a process of systematically collecting, analyzing and expressing data, which will run through the whole process of health education. Community health education evaluation can enable one to know the effect of health education project as well as monitor, control and guarantee the implementation and quality of community health education plan, and thus, it is the key to achieve the expected effect.

（二）社区健康教育评价的内容

Contents of Community Health Education Evaluation

一般社区健康教育评价内容主要有过程评价、近期效果评价、长期效果评价和评价指标（个人或群体），如卫生知识水平、对卫生保健工作态度、卫生行为习惯形成、教育深度和广度、人群健康状况。

The community health education evaluation content mainly includes process evaluation, short-term effect evaluation, long-term effect evaluation and evaluation index (individual or group), such as health knowledge level, attitude to health care work, formation of health behavior, depth and breadth of education, population health status.

第六节 健康教育与健康促进的计划设计
Section Six Planning for Health Education and Health Promotion

一、健康教育与健康促进的计划设计原则
Principles of Health Education and Health Design

对于具体计划的制订，要秉持目标性、整体性、前瞻性、参与性、弹性与从实际出发的原则。

For the formulation of specific plans, we should adhere to the principles of goal, integrity, advance, participation, flexibility and practice.

二、健康教育与健康促进的计划设计步骤
Health Education and Health Promotion Plan Design

按照先对社区需求进行评估，再确定优先项目，然后确定总体目标和具体目标，制定干预策略，最后制定计划实施方案的步骤进行。

The first step is to assess the community needs community needs, and then identify priorities, determine the overall goals, and targets, and formulate intervention strategies. Finally, implementation plans should be made.

（一）社区需求评估
Community Needs Assessment

社区需求评估指了解社区需解决的优先问题，包括社区诊断与流行病学调查，可以通过以下几个途径进行：

Community needs assessment is a process to the understanding on the priority issues. The process includes community diagnosis and epidemiological surveys. This can be done in the following ways:

1. 召开座谈会

Holding Seminars

邀请当地卫生行政部门、爱国卫生机构、预防保健机构、社区管理机构

的领导、专家、技术人员以及群众代表等参加座谈讨论，集中大多数人的意见和基层群众的要求，分析、研究、确定社区的主要健康问题。

By inviting local health administrative departments, patriotic health institutions, prevention and health care institutions, leaders of, community management institutions, experts, technical personnel and representatives of the public to participate in the discussion, it is possible to collect the opinions of the majority and the requirements of the public. Then, the designers can analyze, research and determine the main health problems in the community.

2. 分析文献资料

Literature Analysis

从当地卫生部门、统计部门公布的信息资料、专题报告或发表的调查研究文献中获取有关社区人群健康状况、健康危险因素等方面的资料，分析研究、找出社区存在的主要健康问题。

One can observe the health status and health risk factors of the community population from the information, special reports, or published investigation and research literature published by the local health departments and statistical departments and then further analyze and determine the main health problems existing in the community.

3. 流行病学调查

Epidemiological Survey

发现哪些是社区最严重、最主要的健康问题和需要优先解决的健康问题，并分析哪些行为因素和环境因素是引起这些健康问题的危险因素及其影响最大的因素是什么，特别是行为危险因素在社区人群中分布的情况，哪一类人群受影响最大等，为制定干预策略提供科学依据。

One should find what are the most serious community health problems and priorities, and then analyze what behavioral factors and environmental factors are causing these health problems and their influence, especially the distribution of the behavior risk factors in community and the target population of these risk factors, to provide scientific basis for intervention strategies.

（二）确定优先项目
Priority Setting

确定优先项目指依据对人群健康威胁的严重程度排序，关键在于真实地反映社区存在的群众最关心的健康问题，以及反映各种特殊人群存在的特殊健康问题，决定最重要、最有效的，所用的人力、资金最少而能达到最高效益的项目。

The priority is ranked based on the severity of health threats to the public. The key point is to accurately reflect the health concerns of the community and the unique health problems of special groups, to determine the most important health project with the most influence on public health and highest benefits that can be achieved with the least human and financial resources.

确定优先项目通常需要遵守以下三个优选原则：对人群健康威胁最严重的问题；该危险因素通过干预是有效的；成本低，效益好。

Priority setting is usually determined by following three criteria: the most serious health threat to the population, risk factor that can be effectively intervened, and low cost on intervention with good efficiency.

（三）确定总体目标和具体目标
Identification of Overall Goals and Targets

确定总体目标和具体目标指将最终结果分解为具体可量化的各项指标，包括制定目标和制定指标。

Identification of overall goals and targets refers to breaking down the final result into specific, quantifiable indicators. This includes setting goals and setting targets.

1. 制定目标

Goals Settings

目标是指在执行计划后，预期要达到的理想结果。例如：通过本项目计划的实施，使社区内吸烟人数减少，吸烟率降低，与吸烟有关的慢性病发病率得到控制。

A goal refers to the desired result that is expected after the implementation of the plan. For example, through the implementation of this project, the number of smokers in the community can be reduced, and the smoking rate can be reduced, and the incidence of smoking-related chronic diseases can be controlled.

2. 制定指标

Targets Settings

指标是指目标要达到的具体结果，要求是明确的、具体的、可测量的而又必须达到的指标。一般分为以下三个指标：

Targets are the specific results. A target should be achievable, clear, concrete, measurable and necessary. It is generally divided into the following three indicators:

（1）教育指标

Educational Indicators

教育指标是指要想实现行为改变所应具备的知识、态度、信念和技巧等，是反映健康教育计划近期干预效果的指标。

Educational indicators refer to the knowledge, attitude, belief and skills required to realize behavior change, and reflect the recent intervention effect of health education programs.

（2）行为指标

Behavioral Indicators

行为指标是指健康教育计划实施后，干预对象特点行为变化的指标，也是反映计划中期效果的指标。

Behavior index refers to the change of behavior characteristics after the intervention and the implementation of health education plan, and also reflects the mid-term effect of the plan.

（3）健康指标

Health Indicators

健康指标是指通过健康教育计划的实施，反映干预对象健康状况改善情况的指标。

Health indicators refer to the index that reflects the improvement on the health status of the intervention objects through the implementation of health education plan.

（四）制定干预策略的步骤

Development of Intervention Strategies

一般将制定干预策略分为确定目标人群、制定教育（干预）策略和确定教育场所三个步骤。

Generally, the development of intervention strategies can be divided into three steps: the determination on target population, the formulation of educational (interventional) strategies and deciding on the place for eduction.

1. 判断并确定目标人群类型

Determine the Type of Target Population

人群类型一般包括：高危人群、敏感人群、现患人群以及普通人群。

The population can be generally divided into high-risk population, sensitive population, current affected population and general population.

2. 根据不同的目标人群制定相应的教育（干预）策略

Education (Intervention) Strategies Should Be Developed According to Different Target Groups

（1）教育策略

Educational Strategies

教育策略包含信息交流类（讲课、咨询、小组讨论、科普资料），技能培训类（技能讲座、示范、观摩学习），组织方法类（社区开发、社区活动）。

Educational strategies include information exchange (lecture, consultation, group discussion, popular science materials), skills training (skill lecture, demonstration, observation and learning), and organizational methods (community development, community activities).

（2）社会策略

Social Strategy

社会策略包括政策、法规、规定、奖惩办法。如公共场所禁止吸烟、商店禁止向未成年人销售香烟等政策。

Social strategy includes policies, laws, regulations, rewards and punishments, such as a ban on smoking in public places and a ban on selling cigarettes to minors in shops.

（3）环境策略

Environmental Strategy

环境策略包括如工作场所设立明显的吸烟区、公共场所不设售烟亭等。

Environmental strategies include, for example, the establishment of visible smoking areas in the workplace and the absence of tobacco kiosks in public places.

3. 确定教育场所

Identify a Place for Education

教育场所一般选取在幼儿园、学校、医院、工作场所、社区、居民家庭等实施教育（干预）策略。

Places for health education are generally selected among kindergartens, schools, hospitals, workplaces, communities and residents' families.

（五）制定计划实施方案的要求

Requirements of the Plan Implementation Program

制定计划实施方案要求在项目的设计阶段就要考虑评价问题。对监测与评价的活动、指标、方法、工具、时间、监测与评价负责人等做出明确的规定。

The formulation of a plan for implementation requires that the evaluation should be considered during the design phase of the project. The monitoring and evaluation activities, indicators, methods, tools, time, monitoring and evaluation responsible person, etc., should be clearly stipulated.

三、健康教育与健康促进组织实施的概念与环境

Concept and Environment of Health Education and Health Promotion Organization Implementation

健康教育与健康促进组织实施指按照计划去实现目标、获得效果的过程，实施计划是主体工作部分，也是重点和关键。实施的主要环节有：社区开发、培训、组织干预活动、制定实施时间表、购买和配备必要的物品、计划执行过程的监测与质量控制。

The implementation of health education and health promotion organization refers to the process of achieving goals and obtaining results according to the plan. The implementation plan is the main part of the work, as well as the key point. The main steps of implementation include: community development, training, organizing intervention activities, making implementation schedule, purchasing and equipping necessary items, monitoring and quality control of the implementation process.

四、健康教育与健康促进的评价
Evaluation of Health Education and Health Promotion

健康教育项目计划的评价是全面监测计划执行情况，控制计划实施质量，确保计划实施成功的关键性措施，也是评估项目计划是否成功，是否达到预期效果的重要手段。需要特别强调的是评价不是在计划实施结束后才进行，而是贯穿于计划实施的全过程。

The evaluation of the health education project plan is a key measure to monitor the implementation of the plan, to control the quality of the plan and to ensure the success of the plan. It is also an important means to evaluate the success of the project and whether it achieves the expected results. It should be acknowledged that the evaluation does not take place after the implementation of the plan, but should be carried out throughout the implementation of the plan.

（一）评价的目的
Evaluation Purposes

健康教育项目计划的评价目的有：确定健康教育与健康促进计划的合理性和先进性；确定计划的执行情况，包括干预活动的数量与质量，以确定干预活动是否适合目标人群，资源利用情况是否合理，以及各项活动是否按计划执行；确定健康教育/健康促进计划是否达到预期目标，其可持续性如何；确定项目的产出是否有混杂因素的影响以及影响程度如何；向公众和投资者说明项目结果，扩大项目影响，改善公共关系，以取得目标人群、社区、投资者的更广泛支持与合作；总结健康教育/健康促进项目的成功经验与不足之处，提出进一步的项目方向。

第五章 健康教育与健康促进
CHAPTER FIVE HEALTH EDUCATION AND HEALTH PROMOTION

The purposes of the evaluation of the health education project plan are: to determine the rationality and advancement of health education and health promotion programmes; to determine the implementation of the plan, including the quantity and quality of interventions; to determine whether the interventions are appropriate to the target population and whether the activities are carried out as planned; to determine whether health education/health promotion programmes meet the desired objectives and their sustainability; to make sure whether the output of the project has the influence of confounding factors and the degree of such influence; to inform the public and investors of the results of the project, to expand the impact of the project and to improve public relations for the purpose of broader support and cooperation among the target population, communities and investors; to summarize the successful experiences and shortcomings of health education/health promotion projects for future project development.

（二）评价类型

Evaluation Types

健康教育与健康促进的评价的类型有形成性评价、过程评价、效应评价、结局评价和总结性评价。

The types of evaluation for health education and health promotion are formative evaluation, process evaluation, effect evaluation, outcome evaluation and summative evaluation.

（三）形成评价

Formative Evaluation

形成评价是一个为健康教育计划设计和发展提供信息的过程，包括为指定干预计划所做的需求评估及为计划设计和执行提供所需的基础材料。其目的在于使健康教育计划符合目标人群的实际情况，使计划更科学、更完善。

形成评价的具体内容包括了解目标人群的各种基本特征；了解目标人群对干预的看法；了解教育材料发放系统，包括生产、贮存、批发、零售以及发放渠道；对问卷进行预调查及修改；了解哪些健康教育干预策略适用于目标人群，进行健康教育材料预实验，确定其适宜性；针对计划执行的早期阶段可能出现的问题，根据新的情况对计划做适度调整。

Formative evaluation is a process that provides information for the design and development of health education plans, including needs assessments on designated intervention plans and providing basic materials for the design and implementation of plans. Its purpose is to make the health education plan conform to the actual situation of the target population and make the plan more scientific and more perfect.

The content of forming evaluation including understanding the basic characteristics of the target population; understanding the target population's opinion on the intervention; understanding the educational material distribution systems, including production, storage, wholesale, retail and distribution channels; pre-investigation and revision on the questionnaire; understanding which health education intervention strategies are applicable to the target population, and to determine the suitability of health education materials; modifying the plan according to new circumstances in response to problems that may arise in the early stages of its implementation.

（四）过程评价

Process Evaluation

过程评价指对项目运作情况进行评估。评估内容主要从以下几方面进行考虑：教育干预是否适合于教育对象，并为教育对象所接受；教育干预是否按既定的活动类型、时间、频率加以实施，以及干预的质量如何；教育材料是否全部发放给目标人群，教育的覆盖面情况；目标人群参与是否积极以及不愿参与的原因何在；教育服务利用情况（如展览、咨询等服务项目），以及利用率低的原因何在；是否建立完整的信息反馈体系以及各项记录的完整性、质量如何；在项目实施期间有无重大的环境变化（如各种重大事件），对项目执行的影响如何；工作人员的职业技能、工作态度、责任心及与教育对象、工作人员之间的配合工作情况。

Process evaluation refers to the evaluation of project performance. The contents of the evaluation are mainly considered from the following aspects:

whether the educational intervention is suitable and acceptable for learners; whether the educational intervention is carried out according to the established activity type, time and frequency; whether the quality of the intervention is good enough; whether all teaching materials are distributed to the target population; whether the project covers enough population; whether the target population is actively involved and why they are reluctant to participate; caluculating the utilization of educational services (such as exhibition and consultancy services) and summarizing the reasons for the low utilization; whether to establish a complete information feedback system; assessment on the integrity and quality of the records; whether there is any major environmental change during the implementation of the project, and how it affects the implementation of the project; the professional skills, working attitude, sense of responsibility of the staff and the cooperation between the education objects and the staff.

（五）效应评价

Effect Evaluation

效应评价又称近期和中期效果评价。评价内容为影响健康相关行为的三类因素（倾向、促成、强化因素）的变化和目标人群健康相关行为的变化。

Effect evaluation is also called short-term and mid-term effect evaluation. The contents of the evaluation are the changes of three factors (propensity, contributing and intensiying factors) and the changes of the targeted population's health behaviors.

1. 影响因素

Influencing Factors

（1）倾向因素

Tendency Factors

倾向因素是产生某种行为的动机或愿望，或是诱发产生某种行为的因素。包含目标人群的卫生保健知识，健康价值观，对某一健康行为或疾病的态度，对疾病潜在威胁的信念等。

The tendency factors are the motives or desires that produce certain behavior, or the factors that induce certain behavior. They include the target population's health-care knowledge, health values, attitudes towards a certain health behavior or disease, and the awareness on the potential threat of the disease.

（2）促成因素

Contributing Factors

促成因素是指使愿望得以实现的因素，如卫生服务等客观条件或者实行健康行为的资源可及性。从健康促进角度，有关政策、法规制定情况，行政对健康教育的干预程度也是一种强有力的促成因素。

Contributing factors refer to the factors that enable one to fulfill wishes, inculding objective conditions such as health services or the access to resources necessary for health behaviours, etc. From the perspective of health promotion, the formulation of relevant policies and regulations, and the level of administrative intervention in health education are also powerful contributing factors.

（3）强化因素

Intensifying Factors

强化因素是指形成某种行为所必需的社会条件，主要指第三方因素。如目标人群采纳某健康相关行为时获得家人、朋友或社会支持与反对的因素。

Intensifying factors refer to the necessary social conditions for the formation of a certain behavior, mainly the third party factors. Factors that one receives when a target population adopts a health-related behavior, such as family, friends or social support and opposition, are all intensify factors.

2. 健康相关行为变化

The Change of Health-related Behavior

健康相关行为变化重点关注健康干预前后目标人群的健康相关行为是否发生变化，改变量是多少，各种变化在人群中的分布如何。

The change of health-related behavior focuses on whether the health-related behaviors of the target population change after the health intervention as well as the changing level, and the distribution of the changes in the population.

（六）结局评价

Outcome Evaluation

结局评价是对远期效果进行评价，包括对健康状况和生活质量两个方面的改善情况进行评价，相关评价指标有：

Outcome evaluation is to evaluate the long-term effect, including the improvement of health status and quality of life. The relevant evaluation indexes are:

1. 生理和心理健康指标

Physical and Mental Health Indicators

生理和心理健康指标包括身高、体重、体质指数、血压、血色素等生理指标和人格、抑郁等方面的心理健康指标。

Physical and mental health indicators include physical indicators such as height, weight, body mass index, blood pressure, hemoglobin, etc., and mental health indicators such as personality and depression, etc.

2. 疾病与死亡指标

Disease and Death Indicators

疾病与死亡指标包括疾病发病率、患病率、死亡率、婴儿死亡率、5岁以下儿童死亡率、孕产妇死亡率、平均期望寿命、减寿人年数（YPLL）等指标。

Indicators of disease and death include disease incidence, prevalence, mortality, infant mortality, mortality of children under 5 years old, maternal mortality, average life expectancy, years of potential life lost (YPLL).

3. 生活质量指标

Quality of Life Indicators

生活质量指标是指物质生活质量指数（PQLI指数），美国社会健康协会指数（ASHA指数），日常活动量表（ADL量表）和生活满意度指数量表（LSI量表）。

Quality of life indicators include physical quality of life index (PQLI index), American social health association index (ASHA index), activities of daily living scale (ADL scale) and life satisfaction index scale (LSI scale).

（七）总结评价

Summary Evaluation

总结评价指形成评价、过程评价、效应评价、结局评价的综合以及对各方面资料做出总结性的概括。它全面反映计划的成败。通过总结评价对各项计划的完成情况、对成本—效益等做出总的判断，以总结经验教训，为今后计划的决策提供准确的科学依据。

Summary evaluation refers to the synthesis of evaluation, process evaluation, effect evaluation, outcome evaluation and summary of all aspects of data. It fully reflects the success or failure of the plan. Through summing up and evaluating the overall judgment of the completion of each plan, the cost-benefit and so on, the experience and lessons is summarized, providing the accurate scientific basis for the future plan decision.

思考

Questions

1. 健康教育的方法很多，主要包括哪几种途径？

There are many methods of health education What are the main approaches?

2. 健康促进在推进健康上的主要任务有哪些？请简要回答。

What are the main tasks of health promotion in promoting health?Please answer briefly.

3. 健康传播的影响因素有哪几方面？注意事项有哪些？

What are the factors affecting health transmission?What are the precautions?

4. 请列举健康教育与健康促进的评价类型，并简要说明不同评价的作用。

Please list the types of evaluation of health education and health promotion and briefly explain the role of different evaluations.

第六章　健康风险评估与风险管理
CHAPTER SIX HEALTH RISK ASSESSMENT AND RISK MANAGEMENT

当掌握基本的健康管理知识后，我们需要利用这些知识来进行健康管理，而健康风险评估这项技能是我们必须要学会的。因此，本章节将介绍健康风险评估的相关概念、目的、常用方法等，来帮助大家在一定程度上识别导致风险的危险因素、消灭或控制危险因素，达到预防疾病或延迟疾病发生的目的，从而增进个人或群体的身心健康。

After mastering the basic knowledge of health management, we need to use the knowledge to achieve health management. Also, health risk assessment is a skill we should master. Therefore, this chapter will introduce the related concepts, objectives and common methods of health risk assessment to help you identify and then eliminate or control risk factors leading to risks, then prevent or delay the onset of diseases, thus improve physical and mental health of individuals or groups.

第一节 健康风险评估的相关概念与历史
Section One Concept and History of Health Risk Assessment

风险与健康风险

Risk and Health Risk

（一）风险与健康风险的定义

Definition of Risk and Health Risk

1. 风险的定义

Definition of Risk

风险是发生不幸事件的概率，即指一个事件产生我们所不希望的后果的可能性。某一特定危险情况发生的可能性和后果的组合构成了风险。

Risk is the probability of an unfortunate event, that is, the possibility of the event that leads to an undesirable consequence. The combination of the likelihood and consequences of a particular dangerous situation constitutes a risk.

2. 健康风险的定义

Definition of Health Risk

健康风险是指存在的若干风险中作用于人的身体、影响人的健康的一种风险。具体来讲健康风险是指在人的生命过程中，因自然、社会和人自身发展的诸多因素，导致人出现疾病、伤残以及造成健康损失的可能性。

Health risk refers to one of a number of risks that act on people's body and affect people's health. Specifically, health risk refers to the possibility of disease, disability and health impact caused by many factors of nature, society and development in the course of human life.

（二）健康风险评估

Health Risk Assessment

1.健康风险评估的定义

Definition of Health Risk Assessment

健康风险评估是一种方法或工具，我们用它来描述和预测一个人未来会不会发生某种特定疾病，或者会不会因为某种特定疾病导致死亡。这种分析过程目的在于估计特定事件发生的可能性，而不在于做出明确的诊断。基于评价个人，以问卷方式搜集个人生活方式及健康危险因素信息，完成风险评估分析。针对个人，对由于某一种或几种特定原因造成的死亡或患病风险给予定量的预测或评价。通过提供健康教育或健康咨询服务，能够帮助个人排除一个或多个健康危险因素，进而降低患病或死亡的危险。

Health risk assessment (HRA) is a method or a tool that we use to describe and predict whether a person will develop a particular disease in the future or whether death will result from a particular disease. The purpose of this analysis is to estimate the possibility of a specific event occurring, rather than to make a definitive diagnosis. The risk assessment analysis is based on an evaluation of the individual, using a questionnaire to gather information on the individual's lifestyle and health risk factors. A quantitative prediction or evaluation of an individual's risk of death or illness due to one or more specific causes will be conducted. By receiving health education or health counselling services, the individual can remove one or more health risk factors, thus reducing the risk of illness or death.

2.健康风险评估的深层解析

Deep Analysis of Health Risk Assessment

本书用两个核心概念来进一步帮助理解健康风险评估。

This book uses two core concepts to help further understand health risk assessment.

（1）未来患病或未来死亡

Future Illness or Future Death

具体地说，是要依据循证医学、流行病、统计等的原理和技术，预测未来一定时期内具有一定特征的人群的病死率或患病率。将人群按照健康危险水平进行分层或健康评分，从而评判具有共性的一类人。

Specifically, it is about predicting the mortality or morbidity of a population with certain characteristics over a certain period of time in the future, based on the principles and techniques of evidence-based medicine, epidemiology, statistics, etc. The population is stratified or scored according to the level of health risk, so that a population with common characteristics can be identified.

（2）量化评估

Quantitative Assessment

量化评估是健康风险评估的一个重要特点。其基本思想是将健康危险率的计算结果通过一定的方法转化为一个数值型的评分。比如，患病危险性用患病的概率值作为结果，我们假定0是永生，1是死亡，就可以用0到1之间的数值来评估人们患病的危险性。而且，健康状况不是由单一的某一个方面决定的，健康具有多维性，包括心理健康、躯体健康和社会适应能力。所以，健康风险评估也是全面性的评估，通常从评估确定的健康结果开始，如患病、残疾、死亡，延伸到评估个人的健康功能，如完成日常生活活动的能力、自报健康水平等。

Quantitative assessment is an important feature of health risk assessment. Basically, the idea is to translate the result of a health risk rate calculation into a numerical score by certain methods. For example, using the probability of illness as the outcome of risk of illness, and we can assess people's risk of illness by using a number from 0 to 1, assuming that 0 is eternal life and 1 is death. Furthermore, health status is not determined by a single aspect because it is multidimensional in nature and includes mental health, physical health and social adjustment. Therefore, health risk assessment is also comprehensive, usually starting with the assessment of identified health outcomes, such as illness, disability and death, and extending to the assessment of an individual's health functioning, such as the ability to complete activities of daily living and self-reported levels of health.

3.健康风险评估涉及的方面

Aspects Related to Health Risk Assessment

第一，就临床评估而言，步骤分为体检、门诊、入院以及治疗。第二，健康与疾病风险评估，主要是对人健康状态及危险性的评价。第三，健康过程及结果评估，是针对并发症的预防和治疗的评估。第四，生活方式及行为健康评估。第五，公共卫生监测与人群健康评估。

The first is clinical assessment, whose steps are divided into physical examination, outpatient consultation, hospital admission and treatment. The second is health and disease risk assessment, which focuses on the evaluation of a person's health status and risk of illness. The third, health process and outcome assessment, is an assessment of the prevention and treatment of complications. The fourth is lifestyle and behavioural health assessment. The fifth is public health surveillance and population health assessment.

（三）健康风险评估的发展历史

Development of Health Risk Assessment

健康风险评估起源于美国，其健康评估机构较多、应用广泛。日本、英国和欧洲使用的方法就是基于美国方法的调整、提升后的版本。

Health risk assessment originated in the United States, where health assessment agencies are numerous and widely used. The methods used in Japan, the UK and Europe are adaptations and enhancements based on the US method.

Lewis C. Robbins医生（美国）在十九世纪四十年代首次提出健康风险评估的概念，当时他进行了大量的子宫颈癌和心脏疾病的预防实践工作，从中他总结了这样一个观点：医生应该记录病人的健康风险，用于指导疾病预防工作的有效开展。他创造的健康风险表赋予了医疗检查结果更多的疾病预测性意义。此后，Robbins担任公共卫生部门在研究癌症控制方面的领导者，他主持制定了《十年期死亡率风险表格》，并且在许多小型的示范教学项目中，以健康风险评估作为医学课程的教材及模式进行运用。

Dr Lewis C. Robbins (USA) first introduced the concept of health risk assessment in the 1840s. At that time, he carried out extensive work on the prevention of cervical cancer and heart disease, from which he concluded that doctors should record the health risks of their patients and use them to guide effective disease prevention. He created the Health Hazard Chart, which gave results of medical tests more predictive value for disease. Robbins went on to become a leader in public health research on cancer control, leading the development of the Tables of 10-year Mortality Risk and using health risk assessment as a part of textbooks and a model for medical courses in a number of small model teaching programmes.

到了十九世纪六十年代后期，随着人寿保险精算方法在对病人个体死亡风险概率的量化估计中的大量应用，所有产生量化健康风险评估的必要条件即准备就绪。1970年，Robbins和Hall针对实习医生共同编写了《如何运用前瞻性医学》手册，提供了完整的健康风险评估工具包，包括了问卷表、风险计算以及反馈沟通方法等。至此，健康风险评估的大规模应用和研究发展的基础被奠定。

By the late 1860s, with the application of life insurance actuarial methods for quantifying the probability of individual patient mortality, all the necessary conditions were in place to produce a quantitative health risk assessment. In 1970, Robbins and Hall co-authored the manual *How to Practice Prospective Medicine* for trainee doctors, which provided a complete toolkit for health risk assessment, including questionnaires, risk calculations and methods for communicating feedback. Thus, this laid the foundation for the development of large-scale applications and research in health risk assessment.

自从2000年开始，中国陆续从国外引进了健康风险评估系统。在国内比较成熟的健康管理系统有两个，一个是医博士健康自我管理系统，另外一个是新生代健康风险评估系统。前者整合了国外多个健康管理系统；后者主要是美国密西根大学健康管理系统的引进版。如今，健康风险评估的发展迅速，势头正盛。

Since 2000, China has been introducing health risk assessment systems from abroad. Two mature health management systems in China are the DrMed Health Self-Management System and the New Generation Health Risk Assessment System. The former integrates several health management systems from abroad; the latter is mainly an imported version of the health management system from the University of Michigan. Today, health risk assessment is developing rapidly and is gaining momentum.

第二节 健康风险评估的目的、应用和技术方法
Section Two Objectives, Applications and Technical Methods of Health Risk Assessment

一、健康风险评估的目的
Objectives of Health Risk Assessment

（一）帮助个体综合认识健康危险因素
To Help Individuals Comprehensively Understand Health Risk Factors

健康危险因素是指机体内外存在的使疾病发生和死亡概率增加的诱发因素，分为个人特征、环境因素和生理参数。个人特征与生活息息相关，包括吸烟、酗酒、吸毒、饮食不平衡、职业等，都是影响健康的重要因素。通过对健康状况及未来患病危险性的全面考察，可以帮助个体综合、正确地认识自身的健康风险。

Health risk factors are inducing factors, both inside and outside of the body, that increase the probability of disease and death. They are divided into personal characteristics, environmental factors and physiological parameters. Personal characteristics are closely related to life, including smoking, alcoholism, drug abuse, unbalanced diet, occupation, etc., all of which are important factors in health. A comprehensive review of health status and risk of future illness can help individuals to understand their health risks in a comprehensive and correct manner.

（二）鼓励和帮助人们修正不健康的行为

To Encourage and Help People to Correct Unhealthy Behaviors

修正不健康的行为主要是通过健康教育完成的。积极开展健康教育的核心任务是，促使个体或群体改变不健康的行为和生活方式。健康风险评估在这其中起到了重要作用。通过个性化、量化的评估结果，帮助个体认识自身的健康危险因素及危害与发展趋势，指出个人应该努力改善的方向，有利于医生制定针对性强的系统教育方案，帮助人们有的放矢地修正不健康的行为。

Modifying unhealthy behaviors is primarily accomplished through health education. The core task of actively carrying out health education is to motivate individuals or groups to change unhealthy behaviors and lifestyles. Health risk assessment plays an important role in this regard. The personalised and quantified evaluation results can help individuals recognise their own health risk factors, hazards and trends, and indicate the direction in which individuals should make efforts to improve. It enables doctors to formulate targeted and systematic education programs and help people correct unhealthy behaviors with a definite object in mind.

（三）制定个体化的健康干预措施

To Develop Individualized Health Interventions

健康风险评估可以对个人或群体的健康危险因素进行分析和判断。健康危险因素的多重性决定了健康干预的多方位性，所以我们需要对健康风险评估结果中的危险因素进行详细分析，以便于制定有效而节约成本的健康干预措施。

Health risk assessment can identify individual or group health risk factors for analysis and judgment. The multiplicity of health risk factors determines the multi-faceted nature of health interventions, so we need to conduct a detailed analysis of the risk factors in the results of health risk assessment in order to facilitate the process of formulating effective and cost-saving health interventions.

（四）评价干预措施的有效性

To Evaluate the Effectiveness of Interventions

健康风险评价通过自身的信息系统，收集、追踪和比较重点评价指标的变化，对健康干预措施的有效性进行实时评价和修正。此处评价的是客观实际与预期结果，通过不断地进行比较，找出差异、分析原因、修正计划、完善执行，使健康管理取得更好的效果。

A health risk evaluation is an approach to collecting, tracking and comparing changes in key evaluation indicators through its own information system and to conducting real-time assessment and correction of the effectiveness of health interventions. What is evaluated here is the objective reality and the expected results. Through continuous comparison, differences can be found, causes can be analyzed, plans can be revised, and implementation can be improved, so that health management can achieve better results.

（五）分类健康管理人群

To Classify Health Management Population

根据评估结果，按照健康风险的高低或医疗花费的高低对人群进行分类，并根据分类结果制定不同的健康管理基本策略。这些策略可以用来提高干预的针对性和有效性，通过对不同风险的人群采取不同等级的干预手段，可达到资源的最大利用和健康的最大效果。

According to the results of assessment, we can classify people based on the level of health risk or medical cost, and make different basic health management strategies in line with the classification results. These strategies can be used to improve the targeting and effectiveness of interventions, and by adopting different levels of interventions for different risk groups, the maximum use of resources and maximum effect of health can be achieved.

简言之，健康风险评估目的是把健康数据变为健康信息（信息特指处理后的数据）。健康信息是一个广泛的概念，泛指一切有关人的身体、心理、社会适应能力的知识、技术、观念和行为模式等，可以用来表达人们对健康的判断、观点、态度以及情感。

In short, the purpose of health risk assessment is to turn health data into health information (information specifically refers to processed data). Health information is a broad concept, generally refers to all the knowledge, technology, ideas and behavior patterns related to people's physical, psychological and social adaptability, which can be used to express people's judgments, views, attitudes and emotions on health.

二、健康风险评估的应用

Application of Health Risk Assessment

（一）应用领域

Application Fields

健康风险评估的应用领域非常多。主要有医院、体检中心等医疗卫生服务机构，这些机构会开展个体化的健康教育和健康促进以及有针对性的疾病管理服务。再者，是企业单位等公共场所，这些企业可以引入适合自身的健康管理项目，提高员工职业安全系数，降低员工健康风险，节约医疗费用，提高凝聚力和竞争力。最后，是健康保险行业，健康风险评估有助于确定合理的保险费率，量化投保人群的健康和医疗风险，有效开展专业化的健康管理服务。

The areas of application of health risk assessment are numerous. The main ones are medical and health services such as hospitals and medical examination centres, where they carry out personalized health education and health promotion as well as targeted disease management services. Furthermore, there are public places using health risk assessment such as business units, where these companies can introduce health management programmes tailored to their own needs to improve the occupational safety of their employees, reduce health risks of their employees, save medical costs, and improve cohesion and competitiveness. Finally, there is the health insurance industry, where health risk assessment helps to determine reasonable insurance rates, quantify the health and medical risks of the insured population and effectively carry out specialised health management services.

（二）应用形式

Forms of Application

1. 识别主要健康问题及危险因素

Identify Major Health Issues and Risk Factors

该应用形式通过识别主要健康问题及危险因素，确定健康管理方案，用来分类对待不同的人群。对于处于中低风险的人群，主要是一级预防，包括生活方式和行为的矫正，减少危险因素的数量和降低危害程度。而对于高危人群和患者，优先进行二级和三级预防，通过筛检、系统行为干预和完整的疾病管理方案来防止疾病的发生，减缓疾病的进程和并发症，促进康复。

This form of application identifies the main health problems and risk factors and defines health management programmes that are used to classify different groups of people. For those at low and medium risk, the main focus is on primary prevention, modification of lifestyle and behavior to reduce risk factors and the harm level. For those patients at high risk, priority is given to secondary and tertiary prevention through screening, systematic behavioral interventions and a complete disease management programme to prevent the onset of disease, thus to slow down its progression and complications and then to promote recovery.

2. 评价健康管理效果

Evaluate the Effect of Health Management

该应用形式通常从四个方面来评价：危险因素的控制、患病危险性的变化、成本效果评价和满意度评价。

This form of application is usually evaluated in four ways: control of risk factors, change in risk of illness, cost effectiveness evaluation and satisfaction evaluation.

三、健康风险评估的原理和方法
Principles and Methods of Health Risk Assessment

（一）健康风险评估的原理
The Principle of Health Risk Assessment

健康风险评估是基于评价个人，即以问卷方式收集个人生活方式及健康危险因素信息，对死亡或某种患病的风险给予定量的预测或评价来完成风险评估分析。接着，通过提供健康教育和/或健康咨询服务，帮助个人改变不良生活方式等，进而降低患病或死亡的危险。

Health risk assessment is based on the evaluation of individuals in the form of a questionnaire; it gathers personal lifestyle information and predicts health risk factors, gives quantitative prediction or evaluation of the risk of death or certain diseases to complete the risk assessment analysis. Then, by receiving health education or health counselling services, the individual can change their unhealthy lifestyles, etc., thus reducing the risk of illness or death.

（二）健康风险评估的方法
Methods of Health Risk Assessment

1. 健康风险评估问卷

Health Risk Assessment Questionnaire

健康风险评估问卷内容包括：生理、生化数据，如身高、体重、血压、血脂等；生活方式数据，如吸烟、膳食与运动习惯等；个人或家族健康史；其他危险因素；态度和知识方面的信息等。

The health risk assessment questionnaire includes physiological and biochemical data (such as height, weight, blood pressure and blood lipids), lifestyle data (such as smoking, dietary and exercise habits), personal or family health history, other risk factors and information on attitudes and knowledge.

2. 健康危险度计算

Health Risk Calculation

健康危险度计算有两种方法：单因素加权法、多因素模型法。前期暴露因素指生活方式危险因素（如吸烟）、临床检验值（如胆固醇）、遗传因素

（如乳腺癌家族史）。相对危险性反映的是相对一般人群危险度的增减值。一般人群的危险度是按照人口的年龄性别死亡率来计算的，如果一般人群的相对危险性定为1，那么其他的相对危险性就是大于1或小于1的值。绝对危险性按病种的评估方法一般都是以发病率来表示，也就是未来若干年内患某种疾病的可能性。

There are two methods for calculating health risk, single factor weighting method and multi-factor model method. Pre-exposure factors refer to lifestyle risk factors (e.g., smoking), clinical test value (e.g., cholesterol) and genetic factors (e.g., family history of breast cancer). Relative risk reflects the increase or decrease in risk relative to the general population. The risk for the general population is calculated according to the age-sex mortality rate of the population. If the relative risk for the general population is set at one, then the other relative risks are greater than or less than one. Absolute risk is generally assessed by disease type in terms of incidence, that is, the likelihood of suffering from a disease in the next few years.

3. 评估报告

Evaluation Report

评估报告分为个人报告和人群报告。个人报告一般包括健康风险评估的结果和健康教育信息。人群报告包括受评估群体的人口学特征概述、健康危险因素总结、建议的干预措施和方法等。相对危险性反映的是相对于一般人群危险度的增减量。一般人群的危险度是按照人口的年龄性别率来计算的。

The assessment report is divided into individual report and population report. Individual report generally includes results of health risk assessments and health education information. The population report provides an overview of the demographic characteristics of assessed population, a summary of health risk factors, recommended interventions and approaches, etc. Relative risk reflects the increase or decrease in risk relative to the general population. The risk for the general population is calculated based on the age and sex ratios of the population.

第三节 健康风险评估的种类和注意事项
Section Three Types and Considerations of Health Risk Assessment

健康风险评估的种类

Types of Health Risk Assessment

按功能分类，健康风险评估可分为一般健康状况评估、疾病风险评估，以及疾病风险评估与健康管理策略。按应用的领域分类，可分为临床评估、健康过程及结果评估、生活方式及健康行为评估和公共卫生监测与人群健康评估。

Health risk assessment can be categorised by function into general health assessment, disease risk assessment, disease risk assessment and health management strategies. By area of application, it can be divided into clinical assessment, health process and outcome assessment, lifestyle and health behavior assessment, and public health surveillance and population health assessment.

（一）一般健康评估

General Health Assessment

一般健康状况评估，通常是通过问卷、危险度计算和评估报告这3个基本模块进行健康评估的。但是一般健康状况评估不提供完整病史，不能代替医学检查，更不能代替诊断书，本身不能构成一个健康管理项目，是一种比较基础的评估方法。

The general health assessment is usually carried out through three basic modules, questionnaire, risk calculation and assessment report. However, the general health assessment does not provide a complete medical history. It is not a substitute for a medical examination or a diagnosis, and does not constitute a health management programme by itself. It is a kind of basic assessment method.

（二）疾病风险评估
Disease Risk Assessment

1. 疾病风险评估的定义
Definition of Disease Risk Assessment

疾病风险评估是对特定疾病患病风险的评估，目的在于查出患有指定疾病的个体，引入需求管理或疾病管理、测量医生或患者良好临床实践的依从性与有效性、测量特定干预措施所达到的健康结果以及测量医生或患者的满意度。

Disease risk assessment is the assessment of the risk of developing a specific disease. It aims to identify individuals with a specified disease, introduce demand management or disease management, measure compliance and effectiveness of good clinical practice by doctors or patients, and measure the health outcomes achieved by specific interventions and satisfaction of doctor or patient.

2. 疾病风险评估步骤
Steps of Disease Risk Assessment

疾病风险评估步骤一般包括以下几步：（1）选择要预测的疾病种类；（2）不断发现并确定与该疾病发生有关的危险因素；（3）应用适当的预测方法建立疾病风险预测模型；（4）验证评价模型的正确性和准确性。通过适当的监测方法来进行测评与管理，从而预估人们患病的风险。

The steps in disease risk assessment generally include the followings: (1) selection of the type of disease to be predicted; (2) continuous identification and determination of risk factors associated with the occurrence of that disease; (3) application of appropriate prediction methods to build a disease risk prediction model; and (4) validation of the correctness and accuracy of the evaluation model. Appropriate monitoring methods are used for measurement and management to predict people's risk of suffering from disease.

3. 疾病风险评估的目的
Objectives of Disease Risk Assessment

疾病风险评估的目的区别于一般的健康风险评估，疾病风险评估指的是对特定疾病患病风险的评估（disease specific health assessment）。其主要目的有：（1）筛查出患有特定疾病的个体，引入需求管理或疾病管理；（2）测量医生和患者良好临床实践的依从性和有效性；（3）测量特定干预措施所达到的健康结果；（4）测量医生和患者的满意度。一般健康风险评估的特点对于疾病风险评估一样适用。

The purpose of disease risk assessment is different from general health risk assessment, which refers to the assessment of the risk of developing a specific disease (disease specific health assessment). Its main purposes are: (1) to screen individuals with a defined disease and introduce demand management or disease management; (2) to measure compliance and effectiveness of good clinical practice by doctors and patients; (3) to measure the health outcomes achieved by a specific intervention; and (4) to evaluate satisfaction of doctors and patients. The characteristics of general health risk assessment can also apply to disease risk assessment.

4. 疾病风险评估的特点
Characteristics of Disease Risk Assessment

疾病风险评估具有以下特点：（1）注重评估客观临床（如生化试验）指标对未来特定疾病发生的可能性预测；（2）流行病研究成果是其评估的主要依据和科学基础；（3）评估模型运用严谨的统计学方法和手段；（4）适用于医院或体检中心的核保与精算。

Disease risk assessment has the following characteristics: (1) it focuses on the assessment of objective clinical (e.g. biochemical tests) indicators of the risk of a specific future disease; (2) the results of epidemiological researches are the main basis and scientific foundation for its assessment; (3) its assessment models use rigorous statistical methods and tools; (4) it is applicable to underwriting and actuarial calculations in hospitals or medical examination centres.

（三）生命质量评估
Life Quality Assessment

1. 生命质量评估的定义
Definition of Life Quality Assessment

生命质量评估，又称生存质量、生活质量，其定义多种多样，较普遍适用的定义是：以社会经济、文化背景和价值取向为基础，人们对自己的身体状态、心理功能、社会能力，以及个人整体情形的一种感觉体验。简言之，就是人们对自己生活状态的感受和理解。

Life quality assessment, also known as living quality, is defined in a variety of ways. The more commonly applied definition is a perceived experience of one's physical state, mental functioning, social competence and overall personal situation based on socio-economic and cultural contexts and values. In short, it is how people feel about and understand their state of life.

生命质量是一个内涵丰富的概念，它包括许多内容，如个人的生理健康、心理素质、自立能力、社会关系、个人信念等，指的是人们对自己生活状况的感受和理解。对此概念的理解，会由于人们的文化和价值观念、生活目标、价值期望、行为准则及社会观念的不同而不同。

Life quality is a rich concept that encompasses many elements, such as an individual's physical health, psychological quality, self-reliance, social relationships, personal beliefs, etc. It refers to how people feel about and understand their life situation. The understanding of this concept varies according to people's culture and values, life goals, value expectations, behavioural norms and social attitudes.

2. 生命质量评估的目的
Purposes of Life Quality Assessment

简言之，其研究目的或用途主要在于：测量个别患者及人群的健康状况；定量比较患者及人群健康状况的变化；评价由于疾病带来的负担和对生活质量造成的影响；对治疗进行临床及经济学的评价，选取最佳方案；通过了解生命质量，为卫生政策制定和卫生资源的合理利用提供依据。

In short, the purposes of life quality assessment is to measure the health status of individual patients and populations, to quantify and compare changes in the health status of patients and populations, to evaluate the burden of disease and its impact on life quality, to make clinical and economic evaluations of treatment, and to provide a basis for health policy formulation and the rational use of health resources by understanding life quality.

3. 生命质量评估的特征

Characteristics of Life Quality Assessment

生命质量评估的典型特征是评估现在，不预测未来。评估的重点在体力活动方面，包括休闲活动、体育运动、日常生活活动、职业活动、消耗能量、膳食、精神压力，通过这一项评估，可以识别不健康的行为方式，进而提出改善建议。

The typical feature of life quality assessment is to assess the present instead of predicting the future. The assessment focuses on the area of physical activity, including leisure activities, sports, daily activities, occupational activities, energy consumption, diet, and mental stress. Through this assessment, unhealthy behavioural patterns can be identified and recommendations for improvement can be made.

4. 生命质量评估的内容

Content of Life Quality Assessment

生命质量评估具有综合性，常常是一个主观指标，多采用自我评价。评价结果具有时变性，对健康促进等的效果指标较为敏感，多采用各种量表进行测量，如一般性生命质量调查问卷、临床生命质量测定方法、特殊病种生命质量调查表等。

Life quality assessment is comprehensive; it is often a subjective indicator, and is mostly self-evaluated. The evaluation results are time-varying, and the effect indicators are sensitive to health promotion, which are mostly measured by various scales, such as the general questionnaire of life quality, the clinical life quality measurement method, the questionnaire of life quality of special diseases, etc.

（1）躯体健康方面

Physical Health

躯体健康，是指个人体能和活力的反映，包括活动受限、体力活动适度性、卧床时间等。

Physical health is a reflection of an individual's physical ability and vitality, including limitations in activity, moderate physical activity and time spent in bed.

（2）心理健康方面

Mental Health

心理健康，是指情绪反应、心理感受和意识能力。

Mental health refers to emotional response, psychological feelings and consciousness.

（3）社会功能方面

Social Function

社会功能，指社会交往和社会支持；疾病状况包括主诉、体征和生理测定与病理检查。

Social function refers to social interaction and social support. Disease status includes chief complaint, signs, physiological measurement and pathological examination.

（4）对健康的总体感受方面

Overall Perception of Health

对健康的总体感受，即个体对自身健康状况的评价和主观满意度及幸福感，这反映个人特定需求的满足程度及对自身生活的综合感觉状态。

The overall perception of health is the individual's evaluation of his own health status, and subjective satisfaction and well-being. It reflects the degree to which their specific needs are met and their overall state of feeling about their life.

（四）生活方式评估

Lifestyle Assessment

生活方式评估，也称行为评估。生活方式是一种特定的行为模式，受个体特征和社会关系制约，不健康的生活方式很大程度影响了我们的健康，比如不合理饮食，缺乏锻炼，吸烟喝酒等。

Lifestyle assessment is also known as behavioral assessment; lifestyle refers to a specific behavior pattern, which is influenced by individual characteristics and social relationships. Bad lifestyle greatly affects our health, causing such as poor diet, lack of exercise, smoking and drinking.

（五）体力活动评估

Physical Activity Assessment

1. 体力活动评估的目的

Objectives of Physical Activity Assessment

体力活动评估，其主要目的是评估体适能与能量消耗状况，为健身防病及疾病的辅助治疗提供有益指导，此外，能量消耗的影响因素有很多，包括气候条件、一天中的不同时刻、活动的类型等。

The main purpose of physical activity assessment is to assess physical fitness and energy consumption, so as to provide useful guidance for fitness prevention and adjuvant treatment of diseases. In addition, there are many factors affecting energy consumption, including climate conditions, different times in a day, and types of activities.

2. 体力活动评估的手段

Means of Physical Activity Assessment

体力活动评估的手段选择必须在尽量准确测量能量的消耗水平和完成此评估需要的时间和体能之间进行平衡，借助体力活动日记、体力活动回顾等方法，从强度、持续时间、频率三个角度来评估，但多数依赖于自报数据和通过软件留下的体力活动数据库，这就会导致能量消耗数值上的不准确。

The means of physical activity assessment must balance the need to measure the level of energy consumption as accurately as possible with the time and physical capacity needed to complete this assessment, with the help of physical activity diaries and physical activity reviews, which assess intensity, duration and frequency. But it mostly relies on self-reported data and physical activity databases left through software, which will lead to inaccuracies in the values of energy consumption.

（六）膳食评估

Dietary Assessment

1. 膳食评估的定义

Definition of Dietary Assessment

膳食评估包括膳食能量评估和膳食结构评估，膳食能量评估是对个体的膳食能量摄入情况进行评估，得到不同等级的膳食能量评估结果。

Dietary assessment includes dietary energy assessment and dietary structure assessment. Dietary energy assessment is the assessment of individual dietary energy intake, which can get different levels of dietary energy assessment results.

膳食结构评估是从各种类食物摄入是否均衡的角度对膳食进行评估，分为结构合理、结构欠合理和结构严重欠合理三种评估结果。通过能量和结构两个方面的评估，可以从整体上了解个体膳食摄入情况。根据膳食评估结果和个体基本信息（BMI等），结合中国居民膳食指南，对个体具体的膳食摄入给出有针对性的指导建议，指导建议包括理想食谱和个性化建议。其中理想食谱具有能量合理和膳食结构平衡的特征，个性化建议促进其控制摄入过量食物或增加缺少的食物的摄入量。

The dietary structure assessment assesses diets in terms of balanced intake of various food groups, with three types of results: well-structured, poorly-structured and severely poorly-structured. The assessment of both energy and structure provides an overall picture of an individual's dietary intake. Based on the results of the dietary assessment and the individual's basic information (BMI, etc.), and in conjunction with the Chinese Dietary Guidelines, targeted dietary advice is given to individuals on their specific dietary intake, including ideal recipes and personalized advice. The ideal diet is characterized by reasonable energy and balanced diet structure, and personalized suggestions promote the control of excessive food intake and the increase of insufficient food intake.

2. 膳食评估的目的
Purpose of Dietary Evaluation

古语道："病从口入。"很多时候生病都是因为膳食的不规范，所以通过评估个人及人群的营养状况，给出有益的营养及膳食建议，是很有必要的。根据膳食评估与指导方法设计的个体膳食评估与指导系统，能够让人们方便地对自己的膳食状况进行把握，了解自己的膳食摄入是否合理，并能够根据指导意见调整不合理的食物摄入，使膳食摄入逐渐趋于合理、健康。

As the old saying goes, "Illness starts from mouth." Usually illness is due to irregularities in diet, so it is necessary to assess the nutritional status of individuals and populations and to provide useful nutritional and dietary advice. The Individual Dietary Assessment and Guidance System (IDAGS), designed according to the Dietary Assessment and Guidance Method, enables people to easily grasp their dietary status, understand whether their dietary intake is reasonable or not, and adjust their unreasonable food intake according to the guidance, so that their dietary intake can gradually become reasonable and healthy.

3. 膳食评估工具
Dietary Evaluation Tools

膳食评估常用的评估工具有：食物频率调查表、24小时膳食回顾、膳食日记等。这些工具用来回顾、记录人们的膳食，通过膳食分析来判断人们的状况。

Common tools for diet evaluation include: food frequency questionnaire, 24-hour diet review, diet diary, etc. These tools are used to review and record people's meals and to judge their condition through dietary analysis.

（七）精神压力评估
Mental Stress Assessment

1. 精神压力评估的定义与目的
Definition and Purpose of Mental Stress Assessment

精神压力评估，是科学揭示精神压力与健康结果之间关系的一种方式。

通过精神压力评估，明确自己的精神状况，从而缓解压力，稳定情绪。

Mental stress assessment is a way to shed light on the relationship between stress and health outcomes in a scientific way. Through the mental stress assessment, people can clearly know their mental status, so as to relieve stress and stabilize the mood.

2. 精神压力评估的方法

Methods of Mental Stress Assessment

精神压力评估的方法一般包括心理生理方法、访谈和客观评分法、自报法，其中自报法最为常用。对于个人来说，这主要是从自己的角度对遇到生活事件的性质、程度以及可能的危害情况做出评估。

Methods of mental stress assessment generally include psychophysiological methods, interviews and objective scoring methods, and self-report methods. Self-report methods are most commonly used. For individual, this is primarily an assessment of the nature, extent and possible harmfulness of the life events from his or her own perspective.

思考

Questions

1. 国内比较成熟的健康管理系统有哪些？

What are the mature health management systems in China?

2. 疾病风险评估与一般的健康风险评估有哪些不同？

What are the differences between disease risk assessment and general health risk assessment?

3. 生命质量评估的内容包含哪些方面？

What are the components of quality of life assessment?

第七章　健康保险与健康管理
CHAPTER SEVEN HEALTH INSURANCE AND HEALTH MANAGEMENT

《"健康中国2030"规划纲要》对我国医疗保障体系的发展与完善提出了新的要求，强调推动健康管理与健康保险相融合。本章内容针对健康保险与健康管理展开了系统性介绍，简单介绍了健康保险与健康管理的概念与分类以及两者的关系，并进一步阐述了健康保险的发展现状和未来发展趋势，以帮助大家对健康保险与健康管理有更为全面的认识与了解。

The *Outline of the Healthy China 2030 Plan* puts forward new requirements for the development and improvement of China's medical security system, emphasizing the integration of health management and health insurance. This chapter gives a systematic introduction to the concept and classification of health insurance and health management, explains the relationship between the two, and further expounds the present situation and trends of health insurance, in order to help people have a more comprehensive understanding of health insurance and health management.

第一节 健康保险概述
Section One Overview of Health Insurance

一、健康保险的发展历程
The History of Health Insurance

（一）商业健康保险的发展历程

The Development of Commercial Health Insurance

商业健康保险理念最早诞生于19世纪欧洲的英国。当时英国在全球率先进行第一次工业革命，革命开创了以机器代替手工劳动的时代，以蒸汽机作为动力机，出现了大批蒸汽机器，如珍妮纺织机、蒸汽机车等。然而，大量的蒸汽机车涌现，英国公民缺乏对蒸汽机车的认知，导致城区一时出现多起交通事故。与此同时，医疗技术的不发达让公民在出院后难以继续从事经济活动，生活举步维艰。商业健康保险作为国家福利政策应运而生，提供给这部分公民以保障其基本生活需求。社会的发展使商业健康保险得到不断完善，1930年前后，商业健康保险与国家兜底福利政策正式脱钩，正式独立出现在之后的顶层设计中，并不断完善自身体系。二战后，商业保险作为保障生活有障碍的民众的基本生活需求的一种有利途径，开始在世界范围内飞速发展。它随着社会经济的发展和人们对保险需求的变化而改变，主要受发达国家人口结构的变化的影响。20世纪60年代，发达国家为了控制经营风险的需求，保持经济稳定，以美国为代表，推出管理式医疗保险（MCOs），发展为控制医疗费的医疗保险模式。1973年颁布的《健康维持组织法案》正式明确商业健康保险的内涵、范围、设施框架与基本内容。不仅如此，一大批社会组织也将商业健康保险作为防范自身经营风险的基本手段，如：HMO，PPO，EPO，POS等。商业健康保险在保障民众基本生活需求、防范企业、组织经营风险以及维持国家经济稳定发展等方面的作用显著，已成为国家经济发展中不可或缺的一部分。在我国，商业健康保险起步较晚，是随着商业保险业务尤其是人身保险业务的恢复和发展而开始萌芽的，其标志是1982年上海市人民政府批准的"上海市合作社职工医疗保险"，这是国内首份健康保险业务，随后逐渐出现了不同类型的商业健康保险；进入20世纪90年代，随着经济不断增长，人们对健康的关注逐渐增加，1994年职工医疗保障制度改革在镇江试点，推行社会统筹和个人账户相结合的社会医疗保险模式，至1996年扩大至40个城市，此举促进了商业健康保险的发展；2002年，随着我国《中华人民共和国保险法》的出台，财险公司经监管机构核定可以经营意外伤害险和短期健康险业务，中国商业健康险进入了快速发展的阶段；2006年，国务院颁发了《国务院关于保险业改革的若干意见》和中监会颁布了《健康保险管理办法》，这两个文件的颁布使我国健康保险业务走上了专业化发展的道路。

The concept of commercial health insurance was first born in the UK in the 19th century. At that time, Britain took the lead in the world by carrying out the first industrial revolution, which created an era when manual labor was replaced by machines. Steam engines were used as prime movers, and a large number of steam machines appeared, such as Spinning Jenny, steam locomotive, etc. However, with a large number of steam locomotives appearing in the UK while British citizens lacked knowledge of them, many traffic accidents happened in cities. At the same time, the underdevelopment of medical technology made it difficult for citizens to continue to engage in economic activities after being discharged from the hospital, and their lives were also hard. Commercial health insurance came into being as a national welfare policy and was provided to these citizens to meet their basic living needs. The development of society had continuously improved commercial health insurance which was formally decoupled from the national welfare policy around 1930, and formally appeared independently in the subsequent top-level design, continuously improving its own system. After World War Ⅱ, commercial insurance, as a favorable way to satisfy basic living needs of people who had difficulties in life, began to develop rapidly around the world, and changed with the development of social economy and people's demand for insurance, mainly the changes in the demographic structure of developed countries. In the 1960s, in order to control the needs of business risks, developed countries maintained economic stability. Represented by the United States, the countries launched Managed Care Organizations (MCOs) and developed a medical insurance model that controlled medical expenses. The *HMO Act* of 1973 officially clarified the connotation, scope, facility framework and basic content of commercial health insurance. Besides, many social organizations also used commercial health insurance as a basic means to prevent their own business risks, such as HMO, PPO, EPO, POS, etc. Commercial health insurance plays a significant role in ensuring the basic living needs of the people, preventing risks of enterprises and organizations, and maintaining the stable development of the country's economy. It has become an indispensable part of the country's economic development. In China, commercial health insurance started relatively late. It sprouted with the recovery and development of commercial insurance business, especially personal insurance business, and its symbol was the "Shanghai Cooperative Workers Medical Insurance" approved by the Shanghai government in 1982. This was the first health insurance business in China, and different types of commercial health insurance gradually emerged. In the 1990s, as the economy continued to grow, people's attention to health gradually increased. In 1994, the reform of medical insurance system for workers was piloted in Zhenjiang. The social medical insurance model combining social overall planning and individual accounts was promoted, and it was expanded to 40 cities in 1996, which has promoted the development of commercial health insurance; in 2002, with the introduction of China's Insurance Law, property and casualty insurance companies were approved by regulatory agencies to operate accidental injury insurance and short-term health insurance business, which symbolized that China's commercial health insurance entered a stage of rapid development. In 2006, the two documents, the *Several Opinions of the State Council on the Reform of the Insurance Industry* issued by the State Council and the *Health Insurance Management Measures* issued by the China Regulatory Commission, enabled China's health insurance business to embark on a path of professional development.

（二）社会医疗保险的发展历程

The Development of Social Medical Insurance

德国是世界上第一个以社会立法实施社会保障制度的国家。1883年，德国通过并制定《企业工人疾病保险法》，社会医疗保险正式实施。社会医疗保险作为国家福利政策，在二战后近20年的时间，随着世界经济的复苏，被社会保险水平较低的英国大力推行。1948年，英国政府宣称建立起"福利国家"，1970年，撒切尔夫人实施"开源节流"政策，通过推行社会医疗保险来应对国家内通货膨胀和经济停滞等问题，为缓解福利政策的负担，此举标志着社会医疗保险开始从保障单独人群转为辐射全人群。1989年，德国进行药品价格和药厂补偿的改革，进一步完善了社会医疗保险。社会医疗保险的大力推行，促使亚洲国家也加速了保险制度的改革。我国社会保险开始实施的重要标志是《中华人民共和国社会保险法》的颁布，2010年10月28日第一届全国人民代表大会常务委员会第十七次会议通过了《中华人民共和国社会保险法》，这是一部着力保障和改善民生的法律，对于建立覆盖城乡居民的社会保障体系，更好地维护公民参加社会保险和享受社会保险待遇的合法权益，使公民共享发展成果，具有十分重要的意义。

Germany is the first country in the world to implement a social security system through social legislation. In 1883, Germany enacted and passed the *Corporate Workers' Disease Insurance Law*, and social medical insurance was officially implemented. As a national welfare policy for nearly 20 years after World War II, social medical insurance had been vigorously promoted by the UK, which had a low level of social insurance, as the world economy began to recover. In 1948, the British government declared the establishment of a "welfare state". In 1970, Mrs. Thatcher implemented the policy of "increasing income and reducing expenditure" by promoting social medical insurance to deal with the problems of inflation and economic stagnation in the country, and to ease the burden of welfare policies. This signified that social medical insurance began to shift from protecting the partial population to covering the entire population.

In 1989, Germany carried out reforms of drug prices and compensation for pharmaceutical factories, further improving social medical insurance. The vigorous promotion of social medical insurance had prompted Asian countries to accelerate the reform of their insurance systems. An important sign of the beginning of the implementation of social insurance in China is the promulgation of the *Social Insurance Law of the People's Republic of China*. On October 28, 2010, the Seventeenth Meeting of the Standing Committee of the First National People's Congress passed the *Social Insurance Law of the People's Republic of China*. It is a law that strives to protect and improve people's livelihood. It is of great significance for establishing a social security system covering urban and rural residents, better safeguarding citizens' legal rights to participate in social insurance and enjoy social insurance benefits, and enabling citizens to share the fruits of development.

二、健康保险的概念与分类

The Concept and Classification of Health Insurance

（一）健康保险的概念

The Concept of Health Insurance

健康保险又称"疾病保险"，是指在被保险人身体出现疾病时，由保险人向其支付保险金的人身保险。健康保险的内容主要包括医疗费用、收入损失、丧葬费及遗属生活费等。为防止道德危险，办理健康保险时，保险人通常都规定一段试保期，对被保险人在此时期后罹患疾病造成的损失，保险人方负赔偿责任。其主要的责任划分范畴分为3类，一是医疗费用补偿；二是收入损失或经济补偿；三是残疾或死亡给付。此外，要达到健康保险赔付标准需满足3个条件，首先是疾病必须是由于明显非外来原因所造成的，其次是疾病必须是非先天性的原因所造成的，最后是疾病必须是由于非长存的原因所造成的。

Health insurance, also called "sickness insurance", refers to the personal insurance in which the insurer pays insurance money to the insured when the insured has a physical illness. The contents of health insurance mainly include medical expenses, loss of income, funeral expenses and living expenses of the survivors. In order to prevent moral hazards, when applying for health insurance, the insurer usually stipulates a trial period, and the insurer shall be liable for compensation for losses caused by illnesses of the insured after this period. The main categories of responsibilities are divided into three categories. The first is compensation for medical expenses. The second is loss of income or economic compensation. The third is disability or death payment. In addition, three conditions must be met to achieve health insurance. First, the disease must be caused by clearly non-exogenous reasons. Secondly, the disease must be caused by non-congenital causes. Finally, the disease must be caused by non- permanent reasons.

（二）健康保险的分类

Classification of Health Insurance

按保险性质可以将健康保险分为社会医疗保险和商业健康保险。

According to the nature of insurance, health insurance can be divided into social medical insurance and commercial health insurance.

1. 社会医疗保险

Social Medical Insurance

（1）概念

Concept

社会医疗保险是社会保险的一部分，又可以称为"疾病社会保险"或"健康社会保险"。顾名思义，就是对由于疾病、受伤等原因而产生的医疗费和健康照顾费用给予一定的经济补偿。社会医疗保险是根据国家相关的法律法规而制定的一种社会保障制度，因此具有一定的强制性。不同国家的社会医疗保险体系也不同，我国社会医疗保险体系主要包含三个层次：基本医疗保险和大病医疗补助、企业补充医疗保险和个人补充医疗保险。

Social medical insurance is a part of social insurance, it can also be called "sickness social insurance" or "health social insurance". As the name implies, it is to give certain financial compensation to medical expenses and health care expenses incurred by diseases, injuries and so on. Social medical insurance is a social security system formulated in accordance with relevant national laws and regulations, so it is mandatory. Different countries have different social medical insurance systems. China's social medical insurance system mainly includes three levels: basic medical insurance and medical subsidy for serious illnesses, supplementary medical insurance for enterprises and supplementary medical insurance for individuals.

（2）分类

Classification

国家规定的医保大致分为三类，职工医保、居民医保和新型农村合作医疗。职工医保即城镇职工医疗保险，居民医保即城镇居民医疗保险。

The medical insurance prescribed by the state is roughly divided into three categories, namely, medical insurance for workers, medical insurance for residents and new rural cooperative medical system. Medical insurance for workers is the same as insurance for urban employees, and medical insurance for residents is the same as medical insurance for urban residents.

城镇职工医疗保险：城镇职工医疗保险是最广泛的医疗保险，也就是人们常说的"五险一金"，一般情况下由用人单位与受雇者按照一定的比例共同支付，城镇职工医疗保险能够为劳动者补偿因为疾病而造成的经济损失。

Medical insurance for workers, the most widely-known medical insurance, refers to the "five insurances and one housing fund". Under normal circumstances, the employer and the employee jointly pay according to a certain ratio. It can compensate workers for economic losses caused by illness.

城镇居民医疗保险：城镇居民医疗保险就是给未参加城镇职工医疗保险的未成年人或没有正式工作的居民提供医疗保障。

Medical insurance for urban residents is to provide medical insurance for minors who have not participated in the urban employee medical insurance or residents without formal employment.

新型农村合作医疗保险：新型农村医疗保险就是人们常说的"新农合"，主要由政府出资支持，农民可以自愿参加，要求必须是农村户口才可以参加。

New rural cooperative medical insurance is mainly funded by the government. Farmers can participate voluntarily, but they must be registered as rural residents.

2.商业健康保险

Commercial Health Insurance

（1）概念

Concept

商业健康保险是被保险人自愿参加，由商业保险公司提供的健康保险保障形式。

Commercial health insurance is a form of health insurance provided by commercial insurance companies and participated voluntarily by the insured.

（2）分类

Classification

商业健康保险可通过多种方式进行分类。一是按给付方式划分可分为3类：给付型、报销型、津贴型。

Commercial health insurance can be classified in many ways. According to the payment, it can be divided into three categories: defined-benefit, reimbursement, and allowance.

① 给付型

Defined-benefit

给付型商业健康保险以疾病发生为条件，只要被保险人在罹患保险合同约定的疾病或发生合同约定的情况时，保险公司就要按照合同所规定的保额进行一次性赔付，与实际的花费没有关系。给付型多见于各保险公司的重大疾病保险。

Defined-benefit commercial health insurance is conditional on the occurrence of illness; as long as the insured suffers from the illness or conditions agreed in the insurance contract, the insurance company shall make a one-off payment according to the amount of insurance specified in the contract, which has nothing to do with the actual expenses. It is common in the critical illness insurance of various insurance companies.

② 报销型

Reimbursement

报销型商业健康保险是以发生意外或住院医疗为条件，保险公司根据被保险人在住院结束后所提供的实际支出的各项医疗费用发票，按保险合同约定的比例进行报销。报销型多见于住院医疗保险、意外伤害医疗保险等。

Reimbursement-type commercial health insurance is based on the condition of accident or hospitalization; the insurance company will reimburse according to the proportion agreed in the insurance contract, and the insured should provide the invoices of actual expenditures of the medical expenses after the completion of the hospitalization. It is common in hospital medical insurance, accidental injury medical insurance, etc.

③ 津贴型

Allowance

津贴型商业健康保险是保险公司根据保险合同，按照住院天数、次数或手术项目进行相应补贴的一种保险，可以在不同保险公司购买并重复使用。例如住院医疗补贴保险、住院安心保险等。

Allowance-type commercial health insurance means that the insurance company provides corresponding subsidies contract according to the length of stay, hospitalization frequency or surgical items based on insurance contract; it can be purchased and reused by different insurance companies. For example, hospitalization medical subsidy insurance, hospitalization relief insurance, etc.

二是按保障范围主要分为4类：疾病保险、医疗保险、失能收入损失保险、护理保险。

According to the coverage of protection, commercial health insurance is divided into four categories: sickness insurance, medical insurance, disability income insurance, and care insurance.

④ 疾病保险

Sickness Insurance

疾病保险是以发生约定疾病为给付保险金条件的保险。

Sickness insurance is an insurance that requires the occurrence of a contracted illness as a condition for payment of insurance money.

⑤医疗保险

Medical Insurance

医疗保险即医疗费保险，是对被保险人在接受医疗服务时发生的费用进行补偿的保险。

Medical insurance is medical expense insurance that compensates for the expenses incurred by the insurer when receiving medical services.

⑥失能收入损失保险

Disability Income Insurance

失能收入损失保险是因疾病或意外伤害导致工作能力丧失给付保险金的保险。

Disability income insurance is an insurance for the inability to work due to illness or accidental injury.

⑦护理保险

Care Insurance

护理保险是以因发生约定的日常生活能力障碍导致需要护理行为为给付保险金条件的保险。

Care insurance is an insurance that requires nursing care as a condition for payment of insurance benefits due to the occurrence of an agreed obstacle in the ability of daily living.

三、健康保险的原理与方法

Principles and Methods of Health insurance

健康保险是国家保障公众正常生活的一种福利制度，因此其受到社会制度、社会环境、经济发展状况、人们的需求等多种因素影响。

Health insurance is a kind of welfare that the country guarantees the normal life of the public, so it is affected by many factors such as social system, social environment, economic development status, people's needs and so on.

（一）商业健康保险的原理与方法

Principles and Methods of Commercial Health Insurance

商业健康保险在进行参保额度设计时，往往会考虑到保险标的、保险责任、保险费率、保险金额、保险期限，并将其进行排列组合以满足消费者的需求。商业健康保险具有以下原则：市场、简明、互补和平衡。其主要涉及投保范围、保险责任、责任免除、保险期间、续保、保险费、投保人解除合同的处理、核保、理赔等要素。商业健康保险的精算工作主要由费率制定、赔付率计算和准备金提取几个阶段组成。费率制定阶段即我们通常说的"定价"，是保险经营管理的基础工作之一。在维持商业健康保险方面，主要采取的是保费收入约等于赔款支出，以此来保障参保人。因此，等价和公平是每个商业健康保险费率制定的基本原则。

As for commercial health insurance, the insurance object, insurance liability, insurance rate, insurance amount, and insurance period are usually taken into account and arranged by companies to meet consumers' need when companies design the insurance limits. There are some principles of commercial health insurance, including market, simplicity, complementarity and balance. It mainly involves elements such as the scope of insurance, insurance liability, exemption of liability, insurance period, renewal, insurance premium, the processing of the insured's termination of the contract, underwriting, and settlement of claims. The actuarial work of commercial health insurance mainly consists of several stages: rate formulation, loss rate calculation and reserve withdrawal. The rate-setting stage, which is usually called "pricing", is one of the basic tasks of insurance management. In terms of maintaining commercial health insurance, it is mainly adopted that the premium income is approximately equal to the indemnity expenditure to protect the insured. Therefore, equivalence and fairness are the basic principles of each commercial health insurance rate.

（二）社会医疗保险的原理与方法

Principles and Methods of Social Medical Insurance

社会医疗保险是国家的福利政策，因而该保险遵循"强制性、互补性和补偿性"的投险原则，资金一般都来自政府的专项保险费收入，基金按照"现收现付"原则筹集，按"以收定支、收支平衡"原则支付，权利和义务统一，与就业和收入相关联，保障人群始于部分产业工人，止于全体社会成员，依法设立社会化管理的医疗保险机构作为"第三方支付"组织，其待遇水平决定于医疗保险基金的支付能力。与此同时，社会医疗保险的主要范围是国家强推动下的强制实施，资金主要来自有收入人群的医疗保险费。社会医疗保险主要可以用于支付包括医疗服务的范围及达到医疗保险金支付的标准的机构，民众在支付时将通过档案管理，由社会化管理的医疗保险机构作为"第三方支付"组织进行第三方支付。

Social medical insurance is a national welfare policy. Therefore, the insurance complies with the insurance principle of "compulsory, complementary and compensatory". The funds are generally derived from the government's special insurance premium income, and the fund is raised in accordance with the principle of "pay as you go", and paid according to the principle of "revenue decides expenditure, keep the balance of income and expenditure", with the unity of rights and obligations and relation with employment and income. The protection of the population starts with some industrial workers and ends with all members of society, and a socially managed medical insurance is established in accordance with the law as a "third-party payment" organization. The level of benefits depends on the payment capacity of the medical insurance fund. At the same time, the main scope of social medical insurance is the mandatory implementation under the strong promotion of the state, and the funds mainly come from the medical insurance premiums of income groups. Social medical insurance can be mainly used to pay for institutions that include the scope of medical services and meet the standards of medical insurance payment. When paying, the public will use the medical insurance institution managed by socialization through file management as a "third-party payment" organization for third-party payment paid.

四、构成健康保险的条件

The Conditions that Health Insurance Take Effect

构成健康保险所指的疾病必须满足以下三个条件：

第一，疾病必须是由于明显非外来原因所造成的。

第二，疾病必须是非先天性的原因所造成的。

第三，疾病必须是由于非长存的原因所造成的。

The diseases that will make health take offect must meet the following three conditions:

First, the disease must be caused by clearly non-exogenous reasons.

Secondly, the disease must be caused by non-congenital causes.

Finally, the disease must be caused by non-permanent reasons.

第二节 我国健康保险的现状和发展趋势
Section Two Present Situation and Trends of Health Insurance in China

虽然早在20世纪初期我国健康保险就已开始发展，但是我国当前健康保险仍处于初级阶段，保险所展开的业务规模与覆盖人群还偏少，改革开放40年以来，我国初步形成了以基本医疗保障为主，商业健康保险为补充，覆盖城乡局面的多层次医疗保险体系。

Although as early as the beginning of the 20th century, insurance in our country has started to develop, the current health insurance in China is still in the primary stage, so the business scale of health insurance is small and people involved are few. Since 40 years of reform and opening-up, China has initially formed a multi-level medical insurance system covering urban and rural areas with basic medical insurance as the center and commercial health insurance as the supplement.

一、我国商业健康保险的现状及发展趋势

The Present Situation and Developing Trend of Commercial Health Insurance in China

（一）现状

The Present Situation

我国商业健康保险起步较晚，现在仍处于传统保险向新型保险过渡的阶段，在我国医疗体系中仍然充当着"补充"的角色。随着我国医疗体制深化改革，国家相关文件的颁布给予了商业健康保险的大力支持，商业健康保险作为我国医疗体制体系的重要组成部分，发展迅速，呈现出种类多、保费增长较快的特点；但在现在发展过程中仍然存在着一些亟待完善的问题，如商业健康保险经营主体混杂，权责不清；商业健康保险供需不平衡，商业健康保险的种类不能满足人们日益增长的需求，以及保额较高，缺少保障等；商业健康保险发展所需的专业人才、医疗队伍等软硬件设施不足。

Commercial health insurance in China started relatively late. It is still in the stage of transition from traditional insurance to new types of insurance, and still plays a "supplementary" role in China's medical system. With the deepening of reform of China's medical system, the promulgation of relevant national documents has given strong support to commercial health insurance. As an important part of China's medical system, commercial health insurance has developed rapidly, showing a wide range of types and rapid premium growth. However, in the current development process, there are still problems. For example, the entities of commercial health insurance is mixed, and the rights and responsibilities are unclear. The supply and demand of commercial health insurance are imbalanced, and the types of commercial health insurance cannot meet the increasing needs of people. Besides, the sum insured is high with a lack of protection, etc. What's worse, the professional personnel, medical team and other software or hardware facilities required for the development of commercial health insurance are insufficient.

（二）发展趋势

Trends

1. 创建"医疗+保险"的新型健康保险模式

Create a new health insurance model of "medical plus insurance"

传统的"保险+医疗"的健康保险模式在一定程度上不能够很好地管控医疗费用，导致健康保险陷入亏损的局面。新型的"医疗+保险"健康保险模式是医疗机构和保险公司强强联合，创建全过程、一站式的服务，有利于形成大健康生态圈。

The traditional health insurance model of "insurance plus medical" is not able to manage medical expenses well to a certain extent, leading to a loss of health insurance. The new "medical plus insurance" model is a powerful combination of medical institutions and insurance corporations to create a full-process and provide one-stop service, which is conducive to the formation of a big health industry ecosystem.

2. 发展健康保险种类，保证供需平衡

Extend Categories of Health Insurance to Ensure a Balance Between Supply and Demand

目前，大多数健康保险以给付型保险即重大疾病保险为主，但调查研究表示越来越多中高阶层的人对报销型商业医疗保险的需求日益增长，希望通过增加报销型商业保险为家人全生命周期、全健康领域的医疗费用进行补偿，但我国目前消费型健康保险较为匮乏，因此保险公司应大力发展健康保险种类，以满足不同层次人群对健康保险的需求。

At present, most health insurance is predominantly based on benefit, that is, critical illness insurance. However, research shows that more and more middle-to-high class people are increasingly concerned about reimbursement-based commercial medical insurance, hoping to increase reimbursement-based commercial insurance for the whole life cycle of their families and compensate for medical expenses in the entire health field. As China's current consumer health insurance is relatively scarce, insurance companies should vigorously develop health insurance types to meet the needs of different levels of people for health insurance.

3. 商业保险与健康服务业合作形成大健康产业

Commercial Insurance and Health Service Industry Cooperate to Form a Big Health Industry

大健康产业是一个产业集群，即与健康有关的医药公司、保险公司、医疗机构及养老机构等融合发展，形成一个专业的、功能齐全的健康体系。健康保险可以与体检、医疗和护理等机构的健康服务有机融合，为人们提供健康监测、评估和干预等管理服务，以满足人们对健康险多样化的需求。

The big health industry is an industrial cluster, that is, the integrated development of health-related pharmaceutical companies, insurance companies, medical institutions and pension institutions, forming a professional and fully functional health system. Health insurance can be organically integrated with the health services of institutions such as physical examination, medical treatment, and nursing care to provide people with management services including health monitoring, evaluation, and intervention, which has met people's diverse needs for health insurance.

（三）改善措施

Improvement Measures

问题的呈现给未来我国商业健康保险也带来了改革的方向，具体如下：一是走向专业化经营，打造专业化经营的网络体系；二是构建健康保险经营体系、产品体系和业务经营模式；三是建立销售渠道体系和销售模式，建立风险控制体系和特色服务模式；四是建立专业化管理系统，建立专业化信息系统；五是进一步推动健康管理服务与技术应用以及医保合作关系的深化。

The problem also brings about the direction of reform for China's commercial health insurance in the future, which is as follows. First, we should adopt the mode of professionalized business to develop a professional management network system. Second, we should build health insurance management system, product system and business management model. Third, we should establish the sales channel system and sales model and build the risk control system and characteristic service model. Fourth, we should establish specialized management system and specialized information system. Fifth, we should further promote health management services and technology application as well as deepen the medical insurance cooperation.

二、我国社会医疗保险的现状及发展趋势
The Present Situation and Trends of Social Health Insurance in China

（一）发展现状
The Present Situation

改革开放以来，特别是十四届三中全会的召开，会议提出将建立社会保障制度作为经济体制改革的内容和目标，我国有步骤地进行了以养老、医疗、失业为重点的社会保障制度改革，出台了一系列有关养老、失业、职工医疗等方面的暂行规定，并在全国陆续选定了若干城市作为试点，以积累经验、发现问题，为全国性推广奠定基础。在此基础上，国家又决定逐步提高各地社会统筹的层次，从市县级统筹逐步过渡到省级统筹。由此可见，经过几年的改革，我国社会医疗保险的来源和筹措方式目前正处在新旧交替的特殊阶段。一方面，旧的传统计划经济体制下的资金筹措模式已经渐渐解体，而另一方面新的适应市场经济体制要求的筹资方式还刚刚起步。现阶段我国社会医疗保险体系主要存在以下问题：

Since China's reform and opening up, especially the Third Plenary Session of the 14th Central Committee, the establishment of social security system has become the content and goal of the economic system reform. China has carried out a step-by-step reform of the social security system focusing on old-age care, medical care, and unemployment. It has issued a series of interim regulations on old-age care, unemployment, and employee medical care, and has successively selected several cities as pilot projects across the country. These pilot cities have accumulated experience, discovered problems, and laid the foundation for nationwide promotion. On this basis, the Chinese government has decided to gradually raise the level of social coordination in all regions, from city and county levels to provincial levels. Thus after a few years of reform, the source of social medical insurance and means of raising money are in the special stage of the alternation of the old and the new. On the one hand, the financing mode under the old traditional planned economy system has been gradually disintegrated. On the other hand, the new financing mode to adapt to the requirements of the market economy system has just started. At present, China's social medical insurance system mainly has the following problems:

1. 公费医疗制度的基本框架也依然没有实质性变化

The Basic Framework of the Public Health Care System Has Not Changed Substantially

虽然国家不再统揽一切社会保障经费的筹措,但国家和企业的负担仍然很重。国家负担重,除了因为由国家财政支撑的项目如社会救济、社会福利、优抚安置等继续由国家负担外,还因为国家目前还负担着一部分本应由三方共同分担的社会保险费用。如目前行政事业单位离退休人员的离退休费实际上是由国家财政在负担;虽然在"两江"等地进行了职工医疗制度改革,但就全国范围而言,据统计,到1993年末,全国共计有59万户各类所有制企业,8000多万职工和近2000万退休工人参加了退休费用社会统筹,分别占城镇企业职工的60%和退休人员的80%。但就费用的筹集来源而言,绝大部分由企业统筹,个人缴费率还不足1.5%。

Although China is no longer in charge of all social security financing, the burden on the country and enterprises remains heavy. In addition to the heavy burden by the state financial support projects such as social relief, social welfare, preferential treatment and so on, China is still bearing a part of the social insurance costs that should be shared by the three parties. For example, at present, the retirement expenses of retirees of the administrative institutions are actually in burden by national finance. Although in some places the worker medical treatment system has been reformed, in terms of nationwide, according to statistics, by the end of 1993, the national total of 590,000 various types of enterprises, more than 8,000 workers and nearly 20 million retired workers participated in social pooling of retirement expenses, 80% of employees in urban and 60% of retirees respectively. However, as far as the sources of fees are concerned, most of them are coordinated by enterprises, and the individual contribution rate is less than 1.5%.

2. 医疗费用无法约束，导致基金入不敷出

Medical Expenses Cannot be Restrained, Resulting in Insufficient Funds

医保机构与医疗机构各自为政，导致医保机构无法有效地对医疗费用的支出进行约束，出现"小病大治""唯高价药品是卖"等现象，医保费用节节攀升，导致医保筹资的基金入不敷出。

Medical insurance institutions and medical institutions have their own policy, resulting in medical insurance institutions unable to effectively restrict medical expenditures. Phenomenons such as "over treatment with minor illness" and "high-priced drugs only" have appeared, with medical insurance costs rising steadily, resulting in medical insurance financing funds that cannot make ends meet.

3. 地区差异导致筹资不均衡，福利待遇存在明显的地域差异

Regional Differences Lead to Uneven Financing and Obvious Regional Differences Exist in Welfare Benefits

社会医疗保险是一种国家制定的强制性的制度，各区域各政府可以因地制宜制定征收统筹基金，所以交纳统筹基金的比例和计算办法上都不尽相同。各地方财政和企业的负担水平极不平衡，从而社会保障的社会性未能得到充分体现，降低了统筹基金分担社会风险的能力。不同地区经济发展不同，医疗水平也参差不齐，医疗资源稀缺的地区就给其居民看病带来了不便。因为农村居民对社会医疗保险的认识不足，甚至因为经济原因无力支付，使得"新农保"的覆盖面不全，很多人无法享受到医疗保险的待遇。

Social medical insurance is a compulsory system formulated by the country. The governments of various regions can formulate collective funds for collection according to local conditions. Therefore, the proportion and calculation methods of the co-ordination funds paid are not the same. The burdens of local finance and enterprises are extremely unbalanced. As a result, the social nature of social security has not been fully reflected, and the ability of the co-ordination fund to share social risks has been reduced. The economic growth varies with region, and the level of medical care is also uneven. Regions with scarce medical resources have brought inconvenience to residents to see a doctor. Because rural residents have insufficient understanding of social medical insurance, and even unable to pay due to financial reasons. Thus, the coverage of the "New Rural Insurance" is incomplete, and many people cannot enjoy the benefits of medical insurance.

4. 管理与监督手段不明

Management and Supervision Methods Are Unclear

目前我国社会保障基金的筹集主体较为复杂，涉及劳动、人事、卫生、民政、财政等众多政府部门和保险公司。而1998年劳动与社会保障部的成立，标志着社会保障工作逐步走向统一，这一问题也相应地得到解决。

At present, the main body of social security fund raising in China is relatively complicated, involving labor, personnel, health, civil affairs, finance and many other government departments and insurance companies. The establishment of the Ministry of Labor and Social Security in 1998 marks that social security work is unified step by step, so that this problem also will be solved accordingly.

（二）发展趋势

Trends

1. 扩大基本医疗保险覆盖面

Expand the Coverage of Basic Medical Insurance

医疗保险是社会保险的一部分，人人享有医疗保险是宪法赋予的合法权利。从世界医疗保险的发展史来看，无论发达国家还是发展中国家，都在大力推行全民医疗保险。可以说，医疗保险覆盖本国全民是全世界医疗保险发展的大趋势。我国在中共十六届三中全会上提出了"扩大基本医疗保险覆盖面"大方向的决议，并先后推行了城镇职工医疗保险制度和新型农村合作医疗制度，参保人员的范围也逐渐扩大，从在职员工到在校学生，这标志了我国社会医疗保险向全民医疗保险大步前进。

Medical insurance is a part of social insurance. It is a legal right granted by the Constitution for everyone to have medical insurance. From the history of medical insurance, both developed and developing countries are promoting universal medical insurance. It is the general trend of medical insurance all over the world, that is, medical insurance covers the whole nation. The resolution to "expand the coverage of basic medical insurance" was put forward at the Third Plenary Session of the 16th CPC Central Committee. Furthermore, the government has successively implemented the medical insurance system for urban workers and new rural cooperative medical system. The changes of insured personnel from in-service workers to students in school indicate that China's social medical insurance has made great strides towards universal medical insurance.

2. 多渠道筹集医疗保险基金

Raise Medical Insurance Fund through Multiple Channels

我国现行的社会医疗保险资金来源已经发生了改变，由原先的公费医疗全部由财政支付、劳保医疗经费由企业承担向由雇主和受雇者共同承担。但随着物价的不断上涨，医疗费用也不断上涨，受雇者、雇主和财政补贴还是不能满足日益增长的医疗需求。纵观世界，各国筹集医疗保险基金的渠道还是多样的，主要包括：（1）雇主；（2）受雇者；（3）政府财政；（4）福利彩票的收入；（5）烟草和酒类部分税收。随着我国老龄化人的增长，多渠道筹集医疗保险基金是大势所趋。

The current social medical insurance in China is jointly undertaken by employers and employees, which has changed the original situation that all public medical expenses are paid by finance and the medical expenses of labor insurance are borne by enterprises. However, with the rising of CPI, medical costs are also rising. Thus, the payment made only by the employees, employers and financial subsidies cannot meet the growing medical needs. Throughout the world, there are various channels to raise medical insurance funds, including: (1) employers; (2) employees; (3) government finance; (4) welfare lottery tickets; (5) certain proportion from tobacco and alcohol taxes. With the growth of aging population in China, raising medical insurance funds through multiple channels will become a trend.

3. 法定性和商业性相结合

Combine Social Medical Insurance with Commercial Insurance

目前我国社会医疗保险是属于政策性统筹，即法定要开支的工资项目。但社会医疗保险具有局限性，已经不能够满足人们对于重大疾病治疗的需要，就需要用商业保险来补充。随着社会医疗保险的深化改革和商业保险的不断发展，社会医疗保险与商业保险的有机结合，是我国医疗保险制度建设的重要方向。

At present, China's social medical insurance is according to the policy of coordination, namely the legal expenditure of wages. However, social medical insurance has its limitations, which can no longer meet the needs of people for the treatment of major diseases, so there is a need of supplementing commercial insurance. With the deepening reform of social medical insurance and the continuous development of commercial insurance, the careful combination of social medical insurance and commercial insurance is an important direction of China's medical insurance system construction.

（三）改善措施

Improvement Measures

针对目前社会医疗保险存在的问题，我国采取了积极的措施进行完善。如大力对城镇职工补充医疗保险，社会医疗救助，农村合作医疗，进一步扩大社会医疗保险的覆盖范围，合理调整社会医疗保险的缴费比例，完善统筹基金的支付政策，取消基本医疗保险统筹基金的最高支付限额，起付标准也相对稳定，扩大个人医疗账户的使用范围等措施，以期保障我国社会医疗保险良性运转。

In view of the existing problems of social medical insurance, China has taken positive measures to improve it. For example, the government vigorously supplement medical insurance, social medical assistance and rural cooperative medical care for urban workers, and further extend of the coverage of social medical insurance. In addition, we need reasonably adjust the payment proportion of social medical insurance, improve the payment policy of overall planning fund, cancel the maximum payment limit of the basic medical insurance co-ordination fund, stabilize the deductible standard, and expand the use scope of individual medical accounts so as to ensure the healthy operation of China's social medical insurance.

第三节 健康保险行业中健康管理的概述
Section Three Overview of Health Management in Health Insurance Industry

一、健康保险行业中健康管理的概念与分类
Concept and Classification of Health Management in Health Insurance Industry

（一）健康管理的概念
Concept of Health Management

20世纪50年代末，美国最早提出健康管理（Managed Care）的概念，最初的健康管理主要包括医疗机构通过对其客户开展健康管理或与医疗机构签订经济处方协议两个方面，从而降低客户的医疗支出，最终达到降低医疗保险机构赔付成本的目的。现在的健康管理更加系统化，主要指通过信息采集、健康监测和评估、个性化健康干预等手段，从营养、运动、心理、社会等方面对人们进行健康教育，提高对健康的认知，形成健康的生活方式，从而达到预防和控制疾病的产生与发展，达到降低医疗花费和提高生命质量的目的。

At the end of the 1950s, the concept of Managed Care was put forward by the United States first. The initial health management mainly included two aspects, medical institutions by carrying out health management on their customers and signing economic prescription agreements with medical institution, thereby reducing customers' medical expenditures, and ultimately to achieve the goal of reducing the cost of compensation for medical insurance institutions. Nowadays, health management is more systematic. It mainly refers to health education from the aspects of nutrition, exercise, psychology, and society through information collection, health monitoring and evaluation, and personalized health intervention, improving health awareness and forming a healthy lifestyle, so as to prevent and control the occurrence and development of diseases, and then reduce medical expenses and improve the quality of life.

健康保险行业中，健康管理的概念即是保险管理与经营机构在被保险人提供医疗服务保障和医疗费用补偿的过程中，利用医疗服务资源或与医疗、保健服务提供者的合作，所进行的健康指导和诊疗干预管理活动。其目的是为了投入最少而获得最大的健康效益。

In health insurance industry, health management is the health guidance as well as diagnosis and treatment intervention management activities carried out by the insurance management and operation institutions in the process of insurant's providing medical service guarantee and medical expense compensation, by using medical service resources or cooperating with medical treatment and health care service providers. The aim is to achieve maximum health benefits with minimal input.

（二）健康管理的分类

Classification of Health Management

健康管理主要分为两类：一是健康指导类的健康管理，包括提供健康咨询和健康维护两种管理活动；二是诊疗干预类的健康管理，包括提供就诊服务和诊疗保障两种管理活动。

Health management is mainly divided into two categories. One is health management of health guidance, including two management activities of providing health consultation and health maintenance. The other is health management of diagnosis and treatment intervention, including the provision of medical services and diagnosis and treatment.

二、健康管理的特点
Characteristics of Health Management

健康管理是一个全面管理的系统工程，其主要内容包含了对人们健康危险因素的检测、分析、评估和干预，主要具有以下三个特点：

Health management is a comprehensive management process of the detection, analysis, evaluation and intervention of health risk factors. It mainly has the following three characteristics.

（一）控制健康危险因素
Control of Health Risk Factors

什么是危险因素？健康危险因素就是能够促使疾病或不健康状态发生概率增加的因素，包含了可控因素和不可控因素。可控因素主要有：不合理饮食、缺乏运动、吸烟酗酒等不良生活方式，生理指标异常等因素，这些可变因素可以通过自我行为的改变得到控制。而不可控因素主要是指个人没法控制的，如遗传、医疗政策等因素。健康管理的核心就是通过各种手段控制健康危险中的可控因素，从而降低疾病或不健康状态的发生概率。

What are the risk factors? Health risk factors can increase the probability of disease or adverse health consequences, including controllable and uncontrollable factors. Controllable factors mainly include unreasonable diet, lack of exercise, smoking and alcoholism and other bad lifestyles, abnormal physiological indicators and so on. These variable factors can be controlled through changes in self-behavior. The uncontrollable factors mainly refer to factors that cannot be controlled by individuals, such as genetics and medical policies. The core of health management is to control the controllable factors in health risks through various means, thereby reducing the occurrence of diseases or adverse health consequences.

（二）体现三级预防并举
Simultaneous Development of the Three-level Prevention

健康管理的三级预防包含了针对无病期、疾病初期和疾病后期所采用的不同的手段措施。一级预防，又称为无病预防，主要是预防疾病产生的危因素，针对病因或危险因素采取措施，降低未知的综合风险管理，增强抵抗疾病发生的能力，如现在的婚检、接种等手段都是一级预防的形式。二级预防，又称为临床前期预防（或症候前期），即早发现、早诊断、早治疗的"三早"预防措施。二级预防的目的是防止疾病临床前期或临床初期的变化，避免或减少并发症、后遗症和残疾的发生，或缩短致残的时间。三级预防，即治病防残，是临床中的预防，主要目的是防止伤残和促进功能恢复，提高生存质量，延长寿命，降低病死率。在健康管理三级预防体系中，一级预防应该大于其他级别预防。

The three-level prevention of health management includes different measures for the disease-free period, the early stage of the disease and the later stage of the disease. Primary prevention, also known as disease-free prevention, mainly prevents the risk factors of disease. Taking measures against the cause or risk factors to reduce unknown comprehensive risk management and enhance the ability to resist the occurrence of diseases, such as current premarital examinations, vaccination and so on, are forms of primary prevention. Secondary prevention, also known as pre-clinical prevention (or pre-symptomatic), is the "three early" preventive measures of early detection, early diagnosis, and early treatment. The purpose of secondary prevention is to prevent changes in the preclinical or early clinical stages of the disease, avoid or reduce the occurrence of complications, sequelae and disability, or shorten the time of disability. Tertiary prevention is treatment of disease and disability is the prevention in clinical practice. The main purpose of tertiary prevention is to prevent disability and promote functional recovery, improve the quality of life, extend life span, and reduce the mortality rate. In the three-level prevention system of health management, primary prevention should be greater than other levels of prevention.

（三）服务过程循环运转

Circulating Operation of the Service Process

健康管理的核心内容是健康监测、健康评估和健康干预，健康监测包括建立个人信息档案，如健康情况、生活方式、运动习惯等；健康评估主要是基于个人健康信息及健康体检进行量化分析，评估未来患某种疾病的概率；健康干预建立于健康评估之上，帮助人们认识到健康风险，提高健康意识，制订个性化健康计划等。在健康干预之后仍然需要继续健康监测、健康评估再进行健康计划的调整，所以健康管理是一个长期的过程，是周而复始、循环往复的。

The core of health management is health monitoring, health assessment and health intervention. Health monitoring includes the establishment of personal information files, such as health status, lifestyle, exercise habits, etc. Health assessment is mainly based on quantitative analysis on the basis of personal health information and examination to assess the probability of suffering from a certain disease in the future. Health intervention is based on health assessment to help people recognize health risks, improve health awareness, and develop personalized health plans. After the health intervention, it is still necessary to continue health monitoring, health assessment, and then adjust the health plan. Therefore, health management is a long-term process.

第四节　健康保险与健康管理的关系
Section Four Relationship Between Health Insurance and Health Management

一、健康保险对健康管理的需求
Demand of Health Insurance for Health Management

健康保险是一种金融服务，健康保险对健康管理提供了切实可行的路径。健康保险要求健康管理将费用保障与健康服务有机结合在一起，能够使健康保险在组织结构、运行体系、服务模式和风险控制等方面形成统一体系。因此，健康保险能促进健康管理的资源配置与整合，提升健康管理的有序性；健康保险可作为健康管理的战略性市场渠道，提升健康管理的覆盖性；健康保险能够监督、评价健康管理业的成熟发展，提升健康管理提供活动的有效性，最终实现加强健康管理。

As a financial service, health insurance provides a practical way health management. Under health insurance, health management is required to combine expense protection and health service organically, which can form a unified system in organizational structure, operation system, service mode and risk control of health insurance. Therefore, health insurance can promote the resource allocation and integration of health management, and improve the ordering of health management. Health insurance can be used as a strategic market channel of health management to improve the coverage of health management. Health insurance can supervise and evaluate the mature development of health management industry, improve the effectiveness of health management activities, and finally realize strengthening health management.

在发达国家，健康管理已成为以健康保险为核心的健康产业组成部分，许多市场主体同时提供健康保险产品、诊疗服务计划和健康管理计划。我国健康管理活动自2003年开始，卫生部、劳动和社会保障部与中国保险监督管理委员会三大部委，将健康管理引入保险行业。目前，健康保险机构通过多种形式与健康管理机构合作。

In developed countries, health management has become an integral part of the health industry with health insurance as the core. Many market entities provide health insurance products, medical service plans and health management plans at the same time. Since 2003 when China's health management activities started, the Ministry of Health, the Ministry of Labor and Social Security and the China Insurance Regulatory Commission have taken health management into the insurance industry. At present, the health insurance agency cooperates with the health management agency through various forms.

二、健康管理在健康保险业中的应用

The Application of Health Management in Health Insurance Industry

健康管理在健康保险业中的应用主要包括识别、分类、管理以及计算成本效益4个环节，在保障4个环节有序进行的基础上，运用健康管理服务构成的3个要素：核心技术、实施方式、实施内容，从而提供建立健康诊疗风险管控模式，客户健康档案系统，风险预测和干预技术模型等具体内容。随着社会经济的不断发展，健康保险业已经对健康管理的体系构建提出了具体的要求，包括搭建服务支持平台，建立医疗网络平台，建立信息技术平台，建立技术管理平台，以此来完善服务体系，促使健康保险与健康管理的良性合作。

The application of health management in health insurance industry mainly contains the four parts of identification, classification, management and calculation of cost and benefit. On the basis of ensuring the orderly progress of the four parts, through the application of the three elements of health management services-core technology, implementation mode and implementation content, it can provide the establishment of health diagnosis and treatment risk control mode, customer health record system, risk prediction and intervention technology model and other specific content. With the development of social economy, the health insurance industry requires a health management system with specific platform to promote health insurance and health management of cooperation, including service support platform, establishment of medical network platform, setting up information technology platform and setting up technology management platform.

（一）健康保险与健康管理机构的合作模式

Mode of Cooperation between Health Insurance and Health Management Agencies

健康保险与健康管理机构的合作模式分为3种，分别为服务完全外包模式、自行提供服务模式、共同投资模式。健康管理产品呈现2种形态，一是"简单组合"的产品形态；二是"有机组合"的产品形态。

There are three modes of cooperation between health insurance and health management agencies, which are service-complete-outsourcing mode, self-provided service mode and co-investment model. Health management products present two forms, one is the product form of "simple combination", and the other is the product form of "careful combination".

（二）健康管理产品的市场营销

Marketing of Health Management Products

健康管理产品市场营销的保险适合人群界定方法如下。

The determination methed of population suitable for insurance marketeal as health management products is as follows.

1. 主要根据家庭结构进行判断

Judge Mainly Based on Family Structure

购买保险应该根据自身的年龄、职业、家庭结构、经济收入等实际情况，力所能及地购买人身保险，既能够负担得起保费支出，也能够适当转移相关风险。因此将人群分为以下两类：单身一族和有家一族。单身一族（18~30岁）：对于这类人群，买保险可以首选综合意外医疗保险。这类保险费率低，可以针对意外提供高额身价保障，并能够附加意外医疗和住院医疗，有效补充城镇医疗报销不足的空缺。其次，根据自身情况适当选择补充重大疾病保险，转移未来高额医疗费用带来的负担。一般未婚人士在保障类保险规划的支出不超出自己年收入的20%为宜。有家一族（24~35岁）：对于这类家庭，在进行保险规划时，应当从基础开始规划，首先家庭的每一个成员都要有基础医疗保障、重大疾病保障；其次适当地为孩子准备教育年金与婚嫁金（0~5岁是准备的最佳年龄）；最后考虑的就是养老年金的规划（40岁之前准备是最佳的年龄）。当然，保险规划不是一蹴而就的，是根据年龄阶段、收入阶段的不同而不断规划的。

When buying insurance, one should consider actual circumstances such as age, occupation, family structure, income, and buy insurance which can also transfer relevant risk appropriately with a price within one's scope. Therefore, the population is divided into the following two categories, single people and people who got married. As for single people (from 18 to 30 years old), comprehensive accident medical insurance can be the best choice. This kind of insurance has a low rate, and can provide high value protection for accident, as well as add accident medical treatment and hospitalization medical treatment, which effectively supplement the lack of urban medical reimbursement vacancy. Next, they could choose critical illness insurance according to the personal circumstance to transfer the burden that future high medical treatment cost brings. It is suggested that in general, unmarried personage expenditure of insurance program should not exceed 20% of his annual income. People who got married (ages from 24 to 35): for this type of family, when planning for insurance, they should start from the basis. First of all, every member of the family should have basic medical insurance and major disease insurance. Secondly, the appropriate provision for children's education annuity and marriage fund (from 0 to 5 years old is the best time to prepare). Last but not least, consider pension planning (preparing before age 40 which is the best age). Of course, insurance planning is not achieved overnight; it is in accordance with the age stage, income stage and continuous planning.

2. 依据经济收入选择保险种类

Choose Type of Insurance According to Income

经济收入不同，在规划保险时考虑的重点就不一样。年收入100万以下的工薪家庭主要考虑的是人身保障，转移意外、健康、养老、理财方面的风险。年收入100万及以上非工薪的家庭主要考虑的是资产安全（资产的转移，资产的剥离，资产的传承）。

Due to the different income, the key that should be considered when planning insurance is also different. For salaried families with an annual income of less than 1 million yuan, they should mainly consider personal security and transfer the risks of accidents, health, pension and financial management. For non-salaried households with an annual income of 1 million yuan or more, the main consideration is asset security (asset transfer, asset divestiture and asset inheritance).

第五节 新时代健康保险的发展
Section Five Development of Health Insurance in the New Era

一、新时代健康保险的发展背景
Background of Health Insurance in the New Era

一方面，健康保险的发展潜力，要结合健康政策的整体思路去判断。另一方面，健康保险的发展方向要结合当前社会经济的主要趋势去判断。步入新时代，健康保险发展的主要背景至少包含三大趋势。

On the one hand, the development potential of health insurance should be judged in combination with the overall thinking of health policy. On the other hand, the development direction of health insurance should be judged by combining the main trend of the current social economy. In the new era, the main background of health insurance development includes at least three major trends.

（一）老龄化
Aging

随着出生率的降低，寿命的延长，人口老龄化进程加快，再加上随着经济的发展，生活方式的改变，慢性疾病的增多，医疗需求和社会问题日益突出。

As the birth rate decreases and the life expectancy increases, the aging process of the population accelerates. Coupled with the economic development, lifestyle changes, the increase in chronic diseases, medical needs and social problems are becoming increasingly prominent.

（二）消费升级
Consumption Upgrading

随着人们对健康的关注、需求日益呈现多元化格局，对于医疗服务质量和要求也逐渐提高，而医疗器械及药品等成本也不断增加，这直接导致人们在医疗上的花费越来越高，人们无法承受繁重的医疗费用，甚至"因病致贫"，因此越来越多的人会选择健康险来补偿医疗费用。

As people pay more and more attention to health, the demand is increasingly diversified. So people gradually focus on the quality and requirements of medical services. But the increasing costs of medical equipment and medicines directly leads to higher medical expenditures, resulting in many people's being unable to bear the heavy medical expenses. Thus, more and more people will choose health insurance to compensate for medical expenses.

（三）科技进步

Scientific and Technological Progress

医疗技术的快速进步给健康水平的改善提供了有力的支撑，但理论和经验表明，如果不对医疗技术进步的成本与质量进行有效的评估，健康保障体系的经济压力将会进一步加大。从某个角度讲，商业健康保险应该与医疗机构、社保机构等在数据、业务等各个层面展开合作，成为健康管理的实践者，积极引领健康的生活方式，积极组织并参与疾病预防和早期干预，积极推进成本效益，不断提升技术进步。

The rapid progress of medical technology has provided a strong support for improvement of personal health. However, according to some theories and experience, if the cost and quality implications of medical technology progress are not evaluated effectively, the economic pressure on health security system will be further aggravated. In a way, commercial health insurance should become practitioners of health management by cooperating with medical institutions, and social security institutions at all levels including data and business. Then it can actively lead to a healthy lifestyle by organizing and participating in disease prevention and early intervention, while promoting cost-effectiveness, to continuously improve technological progress.

二、新时代健康保险的推进策略

Promoting Strategy of Health Insurance in the New Era

（一）企业层面

Enterprise

1. 增强健康险在企业员工福利保障计划中的地位，通过与商保合作搭建员工弹性福利平台，提升福利水平同时控制福利成本，保持人才市场竞争优势。

2. 为员工购买税优健康、税延养老等政策性保险，提供经济支持与组织保障。

1. Enhance the status of health insurance in the workers welfare security plan, build a flexible welfare platform for workers through cooperation with commercial insurance companies, improve welfare level and control welfare cost, and maintain competitive advantage in the job market.

2. Provide economic support and organizational guarantee for employees to purchase policy insurance, such as personal tax premium health insurance and tax deferred pension insurance.

（二）个人层面

Individual

1. 关注自身健康状况，增加运动投入，获取可靠健康信息。
2. 强化健康保障意识，有意识地去获取和掌握健康保障相关知识。
3. 充分利用健康险分散个人与家庭的健康和经济风险。

1. Pay attention to your health status, increase exercise input, and obtain reliable health information.

2. Strengthen awareness of health security, and consciously acquire as well as master the knowledge related to health security.

3. Make full use of health insurance to spread health and economic risks of individuals and family.

思考

Questions

1. 按照保障范围分类，商业健康保险主要包括哪几类？

According to classification of insurance scope, what types does commercial health insurance mainly include?

2. 健康管理的特点是什么？

What are the characteristics of health management?

3. 健康管理在健康保险中是如何应用的？

How is health management applied in the field of health insurance?

第八章 生活方式与健康管理
CHAPTER EIGHT LIFE STYLE AND HEALTH MANAGEMENT

在当前社会不断发展的背景下，人们的生活越过越好，吃、住、用、行等各个方面都发生了巨大的变化。在饮食上，漫天的垃圾食品充斥着我们的生活，人们习惯于点外卖、吃快餐；在居住上，电梯房的存在使得我们在上下楼都不约而同地选择了电梯；在用的方面，手机等电子产品的使用，各种"懒人神器"的诞生，给大家的生活带来了数不尽的便捷；在出行方面，我们的生活已经无法离开车辆。这些生活方式的变化，改变了我们的身体，让我们变得越来越安静，越来越懒惰，外加生活压力的增大，年龄、性别等因素的差异，各种因素的叠加，最终导致各种疾病悄然产生，影响着我们的健康。

With the development of our society, people's life get better and better, and there has been a huge change in all aspects of life, including food, hospitality, daily necessities and transport. For example, in terms of food, junk food has come to pervade every aspect our lives, and we are often accustomed to order takeaway or eat fast food. As for hospitality, many resident buildings are equipped with elevators and people take elevators upstairs and downstairs. Besides, the advent of "lazy artifacts" and especially the use of mobile phones and other electronic products, has brought great convenience to us. The last aspect is transport. We have been not able to live without cars. These lifestyle changes have changed our bodies, making us more and more motionless and lazy gradually. In addition, the increase in pressure and the difference of age and gender factors have led to the subsequent emergence of various chronic diseases silently that could affect our health.

高血压、高血脂、糖尿病、痛风以及骨质疏松都是我们耳熟能详的慢性疾病，这些疾病甚至就发生在我们的身边。事实上，这些疾病已经严重威胁到中国乃至全世界人类的健康，是导致死亡的主要原因。

Hypertension, hyperlipidemia, diabetes, gout, and osteoporosis are all chronic diseases that we are familiar with, and these diseases even happen around us. In fact, these diseases have seriously threatened human health in China and the world, and are the main cause of death.

这类疾病又可以被称为"生活方式"疾病，因为这些疾病大多数是可预防的疾病。那么这些疾病产生的具体原因是什么？我们对于这些疾病又可以采取怎样的预防措施？在本章中，我们将会针对高血压、糖尿病、骨质疏松症、高尿酸血症以及血脂异常这五种常见的慢性疾病的健康管理进行介绍。

Such diseases can also be called "lifestyle" diseases, because most of these diseases are preventable diseases. So what are the specific reasons for these diseases? And, how can we prevent these diseases? In this chapter, we will introduce in detail about health management of five common chronic diseases such as hypertension, diabetes, osteoporosis, hyperuricemia and dyslipidemia.

第一节　慢性病患者的生活方式与健康管理
Section One Lifestyle and Health Management of Chronic Disease Patients

一、高血压患者的生活方式与健康管理

Lifestyle and Health Management of People with Hypertension

（一）引言

Introduction

高血压是一种常见的慢性病，它可能会诱发心梗等猝死型病症，然而由于高血压症状隐匿，在并发症发生前难以察觉，因此高血压常被称为"隐形无声杀手"。据统计，每年有约900万人死于血压升高。而另一方面，全世界仍有着50%以上的高血压患者对自己的病情并不了解。事实上，通过提高对于高血压的认识并采取恰当的措施，可以有效降低高血压的风险。本节内容将介绍高血压的健康管理，对高血压进行有效的健康管理将极大地改善未来的生活质量。

Hypertension is a common chronic disease, which can cause symptoms like myocardial infarction. However, because symptoms of hypertension are hidden and difficult to detect before complications occur, hypertension is often called the "invisible and silent killer". According to statistics, about 9 million people die from elevated blood pressure every year. Furthermore, there are still more than 50% of hypertensive patients in the world who do not understand their conditions. In fact, by raising awareness of hypertension and taking appropriate measures, the risk of hypertension can be effectively reduced. This section introduces health management of hypertension. Effective health management of hypertension will greatly improve the quality of life in the future.

（二）引起高血压的主要因素

Causes of Hypertension

原发性高血压的形成是一个复杂而漫长的过程，由环境因素以及其他有关的因素共同交互作用造成的，在不同个体间存在较大的变异。

The formation of primary hypertension is a long and complex process that is caused by the interaction of environmental factors, and other related factors. Also, there are large variations among different individuals.

在环境因素中，个人生活习惯与高血压的成因密切相关，如吸烟、过量饮酒等均是血压升高的影响因素。此外，来自精神应激、长期接触噪音与高温环境的影响，也被发现与高血压的发生存在一定的相关性，体重则是另一个血压升高的重要危险因素。

Among environmental factors, personal living habits are closely related to the cause of hypertension. Smoking and excessive drinking are both factors that affect blood pressure. In addition, effects of mental stress, long-term exposure to noise, and high temperature environment have also been found to be related to the occurrence of hypertension while body weight is another important risk factor for elevated blood pressure.

（三）危害

Harm

1. 心脏问题

Problems of Heart

血压的升高会增加心脏的负荷，导致心肌结构和功能发生改变。诸如心力衰竭、冠心病等背后便经常会有高血压的影子。

The increase in blood pressure increases the load on the heart, leading to changes in the structure and function of the myocardium.

2. 血管问题

Problems of Vascular

长期的高血压患者会有广泛的血管病理改变。除心血管病症以外，高血压还会进一步影响大脑、肾脏、视网膜的正常功能。脑瘤与脑梗是较为常见的不良事件之一。

Long-term hypertension patients will have extensive vascular pathological changes. In the kidneys, continuous high blood pressure can increase the pressure of the glomerular capsule, glomerular fibrosis, renal arteriosclerosis, and cause irreversible loss of nephrons and ultimately lead to chronic kidney disease.

总之，高血压所带来的危害是慢性进行性的，并且可作为其他心血管疾病发展的危险因素（如冠心病、心力衰竭、心室颤动、脑血管疾病、外周动脉疾病、主动脉瘤和慢性肾脏疾病等）。这类病理改变并不完全具有可逆性，因此早期控制血压至理想水平是具有重要意义的。

In short, the harm caused by hypertension is chronic and progressive and can be a risk factor for the development of other cardiovascular diseases (such as coronary heart disease, heart failure, ventricular fibrillation, cerebrovascular disease, peripheral artery disease, aortic aneurysm, and chronic kidney disease, etc.). Such pathological changes are not completely reversible, so early control of blood pressure to the ideal level is of great significance.

（四）高血压的健康管理

Health Management of Hypertension

通过适当的健康管理可以降低发病的可能性或延缓高血压的进程。可分别从运动管理、生活管理、指标检测这三个方面进行干预。

Appropriate health management can reduce the possibility of disease or delay the progress of hypertension through exercise management, life management, and index detection.

1. 运动管理

Sports Management

在运动管理方面，高血压患者的运动干预是一种经济有效的手段。世界卫生组织、国际高血压学会等组织将体育锻炼作为预防高血压前期的首要干预措施。体育锻炼不仅有助于控制高血压，还有助于控制体重，增强心脏的功能，降低个体的压力。良好的体重控制、健康的心脏和乐观的情绪都有益于血压的控制。运动后短期内去甲肾上腺素水平可降低，从而抑制交感神经活动，降低中枢神经系统激素分泌，使血压得以降低。长期体育锻炼可改善血管结构，有助于降低心血管风险。但对于高血压患者而言，运动需要注意以下几点：

In terms of exercise management, exercise intervention for hypertensive patients is an economical and effective means. Organizations such as the World Health Organization and the International Society of Hypertension regard high physical exercise as the primary intervention to prevent prehypertension. Physical exercise not only helps to control high blood pressure, but also helps to control weight, enhance heart function, and reduce individual stress. Good weight control, a healthy heart and optimism are all beneficial to blood pressure control. For a short time after exercise, the level of norepinephrine is reduced, thereby inhibiting sympathetic nerve activity, reducing the release of hormone in the central nervous system so that blood pressure can be reduced. Long-term physical exercise can improve vascular structure, and help reduce cardiovascular risks. However, for hypertensive patients, people need to pay attention to the followings:

（1）运动的科学性

Scientificity of Exercise

运动量要循序渐进，量力而行，切勿直接进行大运动量的活动，这样反而会增加心脏的负担。

The amount of exercise should be gradual and according to your ability. Do not directly engage in strenuous activities, which will increase the heart burden.

（2）运动的合理性

Rationality of Exercise

以适量运动、缓和运动为主，提高心肺功能。

Focus on moderate exercise and moderate exercise to improve cardiopulmonary function.

（3）运动强度的个体化

Individualization of Exercise Intensity

因为不同患者患病的原因不同，个体的身体素质也有所差异，所以，应根据个体身体情况选择不同强度的运动，一般强度不宜过大，应以有氧运动为宜。

As different patients have different causes of illness, individual physical fitness is also different. Therefore, exercises of different intensities should be selected according to individual physical conditions. Generally, the intensity should not be too high, and aerobic exercise is better.

（4）选择适合自己的运动

Discipline of Choosing a Suitable Sport

只有适合的运动才能坚持下去，喜欢的运动才能产生持久的兴趣，比如健身气功、太极拳、步行、交谊舞、垂钓、郊游等有氧运动方式。

Only by playing by a Suitable sport can we stick to it with generating long-term interest, such as fitness qigong, tai chi, walking, social dancing, fishing, outings and other aerobic exercises.

2. 生活方式管理

Lifestyle Management

在生活方式方面，建立良好的生活习惯，保持良好的心态，调整和缓解心理压力，创造良好的心理环境，培养个人健康的社会心理状态，正确对待事物，学会适合自身实际情况的心理调适方法，在必要时刻主动寻求心理咨询与心理干预是科学的减轻精神压力的方法，将有利于高血压和心血管病防治。

In terms of lifestyle, you can establish good living habits, maintain a good attitude, adjust and relieve psychological pressure, create a good psychological environment, cultivate a healthy personal social psychological state, treat things correctly, and learn psychological adjustment methods suitable for your actual situation. Actively seeking psychological counseling and psychological intervention when necessary is a scientific method to reduce mental stress, which will benefit the prevention and treatment of hypertension and cardiovascular disease.

长期过量的饮酒会引起高血压，大剂量的酒精先会导致持续数小时的血压下降，但此后血压会升高。据报道，饮酒量减少约80%后，血压可在1~2周内开始下降。对于重度饮酒者，在突然限制饮酒后，血压会升高，但如果继续控制酒精摄入，血压则会逐渐降低。推荐的酒精摄入量为：男性每日饮用量的酒精量限制在20~30毫升，女性为10~20毫升。烟草中的某些物质可短暂引起血压升高，在普通人群中持续约15分钟，但在重度吸烟人群中，这种血压升高的反应可持续存在。有报告称，吸烟者白天的动态血压升高，并常常导致隐性高血压。吸烟同样是许多心血管疾病的危险因素，在高血压的合并作用下，可引起死亡风险的上升。正如前文所言，吸烟与饮酒是引起高血压的已知危险因素，戒烟限酒均有利于高血压的健康管理。

Long-term excessive drinking can cause high blood pressure. Large doses of alcohol will first cause a drop in blood pressure that lasts for several hours, but then blood pressure will increase. According to reports, blood pressure can begin to drop within 1-2 weeks after alcohol consumption is reduced by about

80%. For heavy drinkers, blood pressure will increase after a sudden restriction of drinking, but if they continue to control alcohol intake, blood pressure will gradually decrease. The recommended alcohol intake is that the amount of alcohol consumed per day for men should be limited to 20-30 ml, and for women 10-20 ml. Certain substances in tobacco can temporarily increase blood pressure, which lasts for about 15 minutes in the general population, but in heavy smokers, this blood pressure increase can continue to exist. It has been reported that smokers have increased ambulatory blood pressure during the day and often cause hidden hypertension. Smoking is also a risk factor for many cardiovascular diseases. Under the combined effect of hypertension, it can cause an increase in the risk of death. As mentioned in the previous chapter, smoking and drinking are known risk factors for high blood pressure, and quitting smoking and limiting alcohol can be beneficial to the health management of hypertension.

肥胖是高血压的重要危险因素之一，研究表明，当减重4~5千克时，血压水平会出现显著的降低，同时体重减轻也可以减轻炎症反应和血管内皮功能的异常。超重与肥胖的个体应当减肥，推荐建立并遵循一个无压力的长期减肥计划，减重目标为BMI降低至25以下。内脏型肥胖不仅会引起高血压，还会引起血糖和脂质代谢的异常，并且与代谢症候群密切相关。因此，内脏型肥胖人群在进行体重控制的同时也应该考虑控制腰围，男性应当控制在85厘米内，女性则在90厘米内。

Obesity is one of the important risk factors for hypertension. Studies have shown that when weight loss is 4 to 5 kg, blood pressure levels will be significantly reduced, and weight loss can also reduce inflammation and vascular endothelial function abnormalities. Individuals who are overweight and obese should lose weight. It is recommended to establish and follow a stress-free long-term weight loss plan. The weight loss goal is to reduce BMI to below 25. Visceral obesity not only causes high blood pressure, but also causes abnormal blood sugar and lipid metabolism, and is closely related to metabolic syndrome. Therefore, for people with visceral obesity, control of waist circumference should be considered when weight control is carried out. Men should be controlled within 85 cm and women within 90 cm.

3. 监测管理

Monitoring Management

相关指标的监测管理也是相当重要的。一般人群及高血压患者需要定期测量血压，及时了解病情的进展，以及对干预方式进行及时的调整。

The monitoring management of related indicators is also important. The general population and hypertensive patients need to regularly measure blood pressure, keep abreast of the progress of the disease, and make timely adjustments to intervention methods.

测量血压的方法可选择自我测量或诊室测量，本书推荐自我测量的监测管理方法，因为自我测量是非医学的，且具有便捷、耗费少的优点，只需通过简单的训练和练习即可在家中由自己或亲人协助下完成测量，也在一定程度上可以避免"白大褂效应"。血压测量应在正确的测量要求下进行测量，即被测人应至少处在静息状态下5分钟，测量时尽可能坐位测量，被测人在测量过程中应避免说话或移动，被测人的手臂应与心脏处于同一水平面中。

The methods of measuring blood pressure in clude self-measurement or clinic measurement. We recommend self-measurement as the monitoring and management method, because self-measurement is nonmedical and has the advantages of convenience and low cost. You can be assisted by yourself or your relatives at home through simple training and practice. "doctor effect" can be avoided to a certain extent. The blood pressure measurement should be carried out under the correct measurement requirements, that is, the subject should be at rest for at least 5 minutes, and the measurement should be done in a sitting position. The subject should avoid talking or moving during the measurement. The human arm should be in the same horizontal plane as the heart.

二、糖尿病患者的生活方式与健康管理
Health Management of People with Diabetes

（一）引言

Introduction

糖尿病通常由不健康的生活方式引起，也与遗传有一定的关联。糖尿病的典型症状被称之为"三多一少"，也就是多饮、多食、多尿以及体重减轻。若不重视糖尿病则往往会引起许多并发症。随着我国经济的飞速发展，人们的生活方式与生活习惯发生了质的改变，随之而来的是肥胖率的上升，糖尿病的发病率也呈现了快速增长的趋势。通过健康干预的模式，掌握健康知识，改变生活习惯，避免疾病的诱发因素，可以有效降低糖尿病发生的可能性。而对已患有糖尿病的人群而言，认识其危险因素，可以延缓病情进展，降低严重并发症的发生，降低医疗费用，改善生活质量。

Diabetes is usually caused by an unhealthy lifestyle, and it is also genetically related. The typical symptoms of diabetes are called "three behaviors more frequent and one thing less", and that is polydipsia, polyphagia, polyuria and weight loss. With the rapid economic development of our country, people's lifestyle and living habits have undergone qualitative changes, followed by the rise in obesity rates, and incidence of diabetes has also shown a rapid increase trend. Through the mode of health intervention, mastering health knowledge, changing living habits, and avoiding causative factors of diseases can effectively reduce the possibility of diabetes. For people who already suffer from diabetes helps to understanding the risk factors can delay the progression of the disease, reduce the occurrence of serious complications and medical expenses, and to improve the quality of life.

（二）糖尿病的形成

Causes of Diabetes

1. 血糖

Blood Glucose

糖尿病的典型特征就是长期的血糖升高，即血液中的葡萄糖浓度过高。

在正常情况下,循环中的葡萄糖含量会维持在一个相对恒定的范围中。正常的血糖来源于日常饮食和自身储存。

The typical feature of diabetes is the long-term increase in blood sugar, which is excessive concentration of glucose in blood. Under normal circumstances, the glucose content in the circulation will be maintained in a relatively constant range. Normal blood glucose comes from daily diet or own storage.

2. 胰岛素与胰高血糖素

Insulin and Glucagon

在维持血糖稳定的过程中,有两种重要的激素,它们分别为胰岛素与胰高血糖素,如果两种中的任何一种激素的水平高于或低于理想的范围,那么机体的血糖水平可能就会出现上升或下降。一般而言,胰岛素协助人体内脏与肌肉摄取葡萄糖,辅助转化和利用葡萄糖;胰高血糖素则负责释放人体内储存的葡萄糖。

In the process of maintaining the stability of blood glucose, there are two important hormones. They are insulin and glucagon. If the level of any of the two hormones is higher or lower than the ideal range, then the body's blood glucose may rise or fall. Generally speaking, Insulin assists viscera and muscles in the uptake of glucose as well as in the conversion and utilization of glucose, while glucagon is responsible for releasing glucose stored in the body.

3. 糖尿病的分类与成因

Classification and Causes of Diabetes

根据现行WHO糖尿病专家委员会的标准糖尿病分为四类:Ⅰ型糖尿病、Ⅱ型糖尿病、妊娠糖尿病和其他特殊类型糖尿病。

According to the standards of the current WHO Diabetes Expert Committee, four types of diabetes are: Type Ⅰ diabetes, Type Ⅱ diabetes, Gestational diabetes and other special types of diabetes.

(1) Ⅰ型糖尿病的成因

Causes of Type Ⅰ Diabetes

Ⅰ型糖尿病的形成,主要是由于自身缺乏胰岛素引起的。人们曾在实验中发现许多与Ⅰ型糖尿病有关的基因。而从环境因素方面考虑，病毒感染也会导致胰岛素产出的缺失，引发特发性的Ⅰ型糖尿病。

Type Ⅰ diabetes is mainly caused by lack of insulin. Many genes linked to Type Ⅰ diabetes have been found in experiments. In terms of environmental factors, viral infection can also lead to a loss of insulin production, further causing idiopathic type Ⅰ diabetes.

（2）Ⅱ型糖尿病的成因

Causes of Type Ⅱ Diabetes

Ⅱ型糖尿病是由于机体存在胰岛素抵抗而产生的，胰岛素分泌初期正常，但在胰岛素利用能力存在障碍后，则会出现胰岛素进行性分泌不足。

Type Ⅱ Diabetes is caused by the body's insulin resistance. Insulin secretion is normal in the early stage, but after the ability to use insulin is impaired, there will be a progressive lack of insulin secretion.

胰岛素抵抗其实就是指各种原因使胰岛素促进葡萄糖摄取和利用的效率下降，机体代偿性地分泌过多胰岛素产生高胰岛素血症，以维持血糖的稳定。

Actually, insulin resistance refers to the decrease in the efficiency of insulin to promote glucose uptake and utilization due to various reasons, and the compensatory secretion of excessive insulin by the body produces hyperinsulinemia to maintain the stability of blood glucose.

（3）其他特殊类型糖尿病的成因

Causes of Other Special Types of Diabetes

其他特殊类型糖尿病，包括遗传因素与环境因素两者相互作用下产生的较为明确的一类高血糖状态，包括胰岛素作用的基因缺陷、胰腺损伤等。

Other special types of diabetes, such as the one caused by the interaction between genetic factors and environmental factors, is a relatively definite type of hyperglycemic state, including genetic defects in the action of insulin, pancreatic injury, etc.

（4）妊娠糖尿病的成因

Causes of Gestational Diabetes Mellitus (GDM)

妊娠糖尿病指的是妊娠前糖代谢正常或有潜在糖耐量减退，妊娠期出现的糖尿病。妊娠糖尿病在某些方面与Ⅱ型糖尿病相似。这种类型的糖尿病虽然是可逆的，但未予以及时重视的话会损害胎儿或母亲的健康。

GDM refers to diabetes that occurs during pregnancy with normal glucose metabolism or potential impaired glucose tolerance before pregnancy. GDM is similar to Type Ⅱ diabetes in some respects. Although this type of diabetes is reversible, it can harm the health of the fetus or mother if left unnoticed.

（三）糖尿病的主要表现与危害

Major Clinical Manifestations and Risks of Diabetes

我们常说的"三多一少"就是由于长期的血糖处于高水平状态、胰岛素分泌不足或存在利用的障碍引起的。由于血糖升高，会出现多尿的情况。由于排尿增多，容易出现口渴的情况。胰岛素分泌不足或存在利用的障碍，导致组织无法正常利用葡萄糖，又会造成消瘦、体重减轻，出现容易多食的情况。通常在糖尿病的早期，这些情况不会立即表现出来，但随着后续的发展，情况会逐渐明显，并可导致许多并发症。

We often say that "three behaviors more frequent and one thing less" is a result of long-term high level of blood glucose, insufficient secretion of insulin or impaired utilization. As blood glucose rises, polyuria appears. Due to increased urination, thirst is prone to situations. Insufficient secretion of insulin or impaired utilization will lead to organs's failing to normally use glucose, and will further cause emaciation, weight loss, and tendency to eat more. Usually in the early stage of diabetes, these situations will not show up immediately, but with the subsequent development, such situations will gradually become apparent and can lead to many complications.

单从"三多一少"的症状我们很难清楚地认识到糖尿病的危害，因为无论是多饮多食多尿，还是出现一定程度的体重减轻，似乎都并不具有致命的影响。然而糖尿病的危险在于其所伴随的并发症，这主要分为急性并发症与慢性并发症，可影响多种器官功能，严重损害生活质量。若能良好地控制血糖，其实并发症的危害也是可以控制的。

With these symptoms, it is difficult for us to clearly recognize the dangers of diabetes, because drinking, eating and urinating, or a certain degree of weight loss does not seem to have a fatal effect. However, the danger of diabetes lies in its accompanying complications, which are mainly divided into acute and chronic complications. They can affect various organ functions, and seriously impair the quality of life. Actually, if blood glucose can be well controlled, complications can also be controlled.

（四）糖尿病的健康管理

Health Management of Diabetes

糖尿病目前仍不能根治，但健康管理可以起到一定的帮助。糖尿病健康管理的目的是尽可能地使糖代谢恢复到正常状态，改善胰岛素抵抗的状态。因此，无论对于糖尿病患者还是具有高危因素的人群又或是健康人群，合理的健康管理方式都可以减低糖尿病发病的可能性。糖尿病的健康管理与高血压的健康管理大致相同，也包括运动管理、生活习惯管理、相关监测等方面。

Diabetes is still not cured, but health management can do some help. The purpose of diabetes health management is to restore glucose metabolism to a normal state as much as possible and improve the state of insulin resistance. Therefore, whether for diabetic patients or healthy people, reasonable health management methods can reduce the possibility of diabetes. The health management of diabetes is roughly the same as the health management of hypertension, which also includes exercise management, lifestyle management, and related monitoring.

1. 运动管理

Exercise Management

运动管理在糖尿病管理中占据着重要的地位，这点对Ⅱ型糖尿病患者而言尤为重要。有证据表明：运动有助于控制血糖和体重，运动对改善心血管健康的益处同样使Ⅰ型糖尿病患者受益。具体的运动管理方案需要根据年龄、性别、糖尿病类型、有无并发症等综合考虑，需要注意以下几点：

Exercise management occupies an important position in diabetes management, which is particularly important for patients with Type Ⅱ diabetes. There is evidence that exercise can help control blood glucose and weight. The benefits of exercise for improving cardiovascular health also benefit patients with Type Ⅰ diabetes. Specific exercise management plans need to be comprehensively considered based on age, gender, type of diabetes, and whether there are complications, etc., and the following points should be noted:

（1）运动的科学性

Scientificity of Exercise

运动方式以有氧运动为宜。在Ⅰ型和Ⅱ型糖尿病患者中，中度到高度的有氧运动量与较低的心血管疾病和总死亡风险相关。

Aerobic exercise is better than other exercises. As for patients of Type Ⅰ and Type Ⅱ diabetes, moderate to high levels of aerobic exercise are associated with a lower risk of cardiovascular disease and overall death.

（2）运动的合理性

Rationality of Exercise

对于长时间坐着的个体而言，应该每30分钟进行一次轻微的活动，这样有利于血糖的控制。建议每周进行150分钟的中等强度运动，且运动休息的时间间隔不应超过2天，锻炼时一定要控制运动强度。对于肥胖人群，运动量要适当加大以起到减肥的效果。对于Ⅰ型糖尿病患者而言，需要额外的碳水化合物摄入和/或胰岛素减少，以维持体育活动期间和之后的血糖平衡。

For individuals who sit for a long time, light activities should be performed every 30 minutes to help control blood glucose. It is recommended to do 150 minutes of moderate-intensity exercise every week, and the time interval between exercise and breaks should not exceed 2 days. The exercise intensity must be controlled during exercise. For obese people, the amount of exercise should be appropriately increased to achieve the effect of weight loss. For patients with Type

I diabetes, additional carbohydrate intake and/or insulin reduction are required to maintain blood glucose balance during and after physical activity.

(3) 运动的个体化

Individualization of Exercise

运动项目和运动量要个体化。应将体力活动融入日常的生活中，如尽量少用汽车代步或乘电梯等。

The items and amount of exercise should be individualized. Physical activities should be integrated into daily life, such as using cars or elevators as less as possible.

基于以上的注意事项，运动疗法的原则可归纳为"一三五七法"。即糖尿病患者运动要持之以恒，每天都运动。一次运动不少于30分钟（对于从来没参加过运动的患者，可从每天5~10分钟、每周2~3次开始，逐渐增加）；每周运动不少于5次；运动强度应该以浑身发热、出汗但不大汗淋漓为宜，心率应控制在"170-年龄"，这样运动则有效且安全。

Based on the above precautions, diabetic patients must exercise consistently and exercise every day. Exercise no less than 30 minutes at one time (for patients who have never participated in exercise, start from 5–10 minutes a day, 2–3 times a week, and gradually increase). Exercise no less than 5 times a week. Exercise intensity should be kept at sweating but not profusely. The heart rate should be controlled at "170 minus age" so that exercise is effective and safe.

2. 生活习惯管理

Lifestyle Management

糖尿病患者需要建立良好的生活习惯，注意个人卫生，以避免感染的发生。保持一个良好的心态。有证据表明不良的心态会导致血糖水平的上升。戒烟限酒，烟草与酒精一定程度上会协同并发症的发生，增加不良事件的发生概率。超重及肥胖者应适当减肥，这对于增强胰岛素的敏感性格外重要。

Diabetes patients need to establish good living habits and pay attention to personal hygiene to avoid infection. Diabetes patients should maintain a good state of mind. There is evidence that a bad state of mind can cause blood glucose levels to rise. Both smoking and alcohol should be quitted. To a certain extent, tobacco and alcohol will synergize the occurrence of complications and increase the probability of adverse events. Those who are overweight and obese should lose weight appropriately, which is particularly important for enhancing insulin sensitivity.

3. 相关监测管理

Related Monitoring

对于糖尿病患者，推荐居家进行定期监测血糖。糖尿病患者对血糖进行定期监测，有助于控制血糖水平，有助于树立对疾病的信心，了解现阶段的治疗与生活方式对疾病的影响，减少长期并发症的发生。

For patients with diabetes, regular home blood glucose monitoring is recommended. Regular monitoring of blood sugar for diabetic patients helps to control blood sugar levels, helps to build confidence in the disease, understand the impact of current treatment and lifestyle on the disease, and reduces the occurrence of long-term complications.

血糖监测除在医疗机构中进行外，也可以由个人在家庭中进行自我监测。自我监测可以是在一天的某些时间（比如晨起空腹状态或餐后）也可以是检查一段时间（比如两周）的血糖水平。目前市场上有许多不同类型的居家血糖监测设备，患者只需通过收集少量的血液样本，通过仪器，便可得到血糖的读值。个人血糖监测的频率取决于个人的实际情况，包括了糖尿病的类型等。推荐的监测时间点包括以下几个：早餐前（空腹）、午饭/晚饭前、饭后两小时、睡前、在剧烈运动之前以及当个人感觉不适的时候（可能会是血糖升高后的情况）。

In addition to blood glucose monitoring in medical institutions, it can also be done at home. Self-monitoring can be done at certain times of the day (such as getting up in the morning on an empty stomach or after a meal) or checking blood glucose levels over a period of time (such as two weeks). At present, there are many different types of home blood glucose monitoring equipment on the market. Patients only need to collect a small blood sample to get the value of blood glucose with the help of such instruments. The frequency of individual glucose monitoring depends on the individual's actual situation, including the type of diabetes. Recommended monitoring times include: before breakfast (on an empty stomach), before lunch and dinner, two hours after dinner, before bedtime, before strenuous exercise, and when an individual feels unwell (possibly after a rise in blood glucose).

对于已患有糖尿病的人群而言,除专业性的检查之外,对体重变化、饮食变化等生活上的改变进行检查也有助于第一时间了解相关问题的变化。

For people with diabetes, in addition to professional inspections, inspections for changes in life such as weight changes and diet changes also help to understand the changes in related issues at first hand.

三、骨质疏松症患者的生活方式与健康管理
Section Three–Health Management of People with Osteoporosis

(一)引言

Introduction

骨质疏松症是老年人骨折的最常见原因,常常引起脊椎骨、上肢骨、骨盆等部位的骨折,是一种由多种因素引起的代谢性骨病。严重骨质疏松的患者甚至可能因为打喷嚏而出现骨的断裂。在骨折发生之前,通常没有任何症状,难以令人主动察觉。由于骨折,骨质疏松的人群后期可能会伴有慢性疼痛以及正常活动能力下降。若不予以重视,随着病情的进一步进展可出现脊柱变形和多发骨折等情况,具有较高的致残致死率。因此,骨质疏松症严重影响了患者的生活质量,也随之产生巨大的医疗成本。骨质疏松的发生与年龄相关,随着年龄的增长,骨质疏松症变得越来越普遍。相较于欧美国家,东亚人群更易患上骨质疏松症。然而目前,相较于"三高症"、癌症常见的疾病,我国人群对骨质疏松症的认识相对较浅。通过了解骨质疏松症的健康管理,可以带动身边人群对骨质疏松症的认识,避免不良事件的发生。

Osteoporosis is a metabolic bone disease caused by a variety of factors. Patients with severe fractures may even experience bone fractures due to sneezing.

Before the fracture occurs, there are usually no symptoms and it is difficult for people to actively notice. Due to bone fractures, people with osteoporosis may have chronic pain and decreased normal mobility in the later stages. If not taken seriously, spinal deformation and multiple fractures may occur with the further progress of the disease, which has a high disability fatality rate. Therefore, osteoporosis seriously affects the patient's quality of life, and consequently generates huge medical costs. The occurrence of osteoporosis is related to age. As we get older, osteoporosis becomes more and more common. Compared with European and American countries, people in East Asia are more susceptible to osteoporosis. However, compared with common diseases such as "three high disease" and cancer, the understanding of osteoporosis in our population is relatively shallow now. By learning health management of osteoporosis, we will drive the people around us to understand fractures and avoid the occurrence of adverse events.

（二）骨质疏松症的形成

Causes of Osteoporosis

1. 骨重建

Bone Remodeling

在人体正常性成熟后，骨的代谢主要以骨重建的形式进行。对于一个成年人来说，每年约有10%的骨骼通过这一途径得到更新。当发生骨折或正常活动出现微小损伤时，骨重建会参与骨折后骨的重塑与陈骨替换。

After the sexual maturation, bone metabolism is mainly carried out in the form of bone remodeling. For an adult, about 10% of bones are renewed in this way every year. When a fracture occurs or a minor injury occurs in normal activities, bone reconstruction will participate in the remodeling and replacement of bone after the fracture.

2. 骨质疏松症的成因

Causes of Osteoporosis

与其他灵长类动物相比，人类的骨质密度较低，人类的骨骼多孔性较强，更容易出现骨质疏松症。骨质疏松症一般分为原发性和继发性两大类，原发性骨质疏松症又分为Ⅰ型与Ⅱ型。Ⅰ型原发性骨质疏松症是由于女性绝经后出现激素水平的改变而引起的，故又称之为绝经后骨质疏松症，一般发生在妇女绝经后5~10年。Ⅱ型原发性骨质疏松症又称为老年性骨质疏松症，一般指老人70岁后发生的骨质疏松症。继发性骨质疏松症是由于某些原发病因明确所引起的骨质疏松症。由于继发性骨质疏松症是由其他原发因素所导致的，故在本节中主要针对原发性骨质疏松症的健康管理做介绍。

Compared with other primates, humans have lower bone density and highly porous bones that are more prone to osteoporosis. Generally speaking, osteoporosis can be divided into two categories: primary and secondary, and primary osteoporosis is divided into type Ⅰ and type Ⅱ. Type Ⅰ primary osteoporosis is caused by changes in hormone levels in women after menopause, so it is called postmenopausal osteoporosis (PMOP), which generally occurs within 5–10 years after menopause. Type Ⅱ primary osteoporosis is also called senile osteoporosis, which generally refers to osteoporosis that occurs after one being 70 years old. Secondary osteoporosis is osteoporosis caused by certain primary causes. Since secondary osteoporosis is caused by other primary factors, this section mainly focuses on the health management of primary osteoporosis.

原发性骨质疏松症存在不可改变的成因与（潜在的）可改变的成因。正如上面所说的，绝经后骨质疏松症是更年期后女性发生骨质疏松症的主要类型，既往骨折病史也被发现于骨质疏松症的发病率相关。可改变的病因包括酗酒、吸烟、营养缺乏、缺乏锻炼、过度的耐力训练、过度饮用软饮料、维生素D缺乏等。

Primary osteoporosis has unalterable causes and (potentially) alterable causes. As mentioned above, postmenopausal osteoporosis is the main type of osteoporosis in postmenopausal women. The history of previous fractures has also been found to be related to the incidence of osteoporosis. Modifiable causes include alcoholism, smoking, nutritional deficiencies, lack of exercise, excessive endurance training, excessive consumption of soft drinks, and vitamin D deficiency.

（三）骨质疏松症的危害

Harm of Osteoporosis

由于骨质疏松症一般是指骨密度的降低，因此骨质疏松症本身是没有症状的，因此骨质疏松症也是一种"寂静的疾病"。但随着病情的持续，骨量不断丢失。

Because osteoporosis generally refers to the reduction of bone density, osteoporosis itself is asymptomatic, and therefore osteoporosis is also a "quiet disease". However, as the disease continues, bone loses continuously.

对于早期患骨质疏松症的人而言，可能会出现腰背疼痛或全身性的骨痛，这类疼痛与一般性的疼痛不同的是在于其不具有固定的部位，属于弥漫性的疼痛，体格检查亦不能发现明显的压痛区。除疼痛外，患者容易出现乏力、肌肉力量下降等表现。对于患骨质疏松症的人，他们很有可能在无外伤或仅仅是受到了较微外伤情况下出现骨折，骨折最常见的部位是在胸、腰椎、髋部等部位也可以发生骨折。这类骨折如果不及时处理常常会导致残疾，而急性和慢性疼痛往往归因于骨质疏松导致的骨折。

For patients with osteoporosis on the early stage, low back pain or general bone pain may occur. This type of pain is different from general pain in that it does not have a fixed location, which is diffuse pain. The examination could not find obvious tenderness areas. In addition to pain, patients are prone to fatigue and decreased muscle strength. For patients with osteoporosis, they are likely to have fractures without trauma or only minor trauma. The most common fracture sites are in the thoracic and lumbar spine, other parts like hips can also be fractured. If this type of fracture is not treated in time, it often leads to disability. Acute and chronic pain are often attributed to fractures caused by osteoporosis.

（四）骨质疏松症的健康管理

Health Management of Osteoporosis

从健康管理的角度而言，骨质疏松症的健康管理也包括了运动管理、生活习惯管理、相关监测等方面。对骨质疏松症的易感人群而言，疾病的早期发现，可提高骨质量，以降低骨质疏松症的风险。

From the perspective of health management, the health management of osteoporosis also includes exercise management, lifestyle management, and related monitoring. For people who are susceptible to osteoporosis, early detection of the disease can improve bone quality and reduce the risk of osteoporosis.

1. 运动管理

Exercise Management

适量的运动有助于骨骼的健康。体育锻炼可以有助于增加骨密度，规律运动的人群平均骨质流失率较少，同时体育锻炼也能降低骨折的发生概率。运动还可改善机体敏捷性、力量、姿势、平衡、增强肌肉等，具有减少跌倒风险、减轻疼痛等方面的作用。骨质疏松症患者在运动项目的选择上应当更注重于提高耐受力与平衡能力，这里推荐有氧负重训练或抗阻运动，如散步、爬楼梯、慢跑和太极等，有较多的证据表明了有氧负重项目的运动员相较于自行车、游泳等无负重的运动员表现出了更高的骨密度。

Appropriate exercise contributes to bone health. Exercise can help increase bone density, and the average bone loss rate of people who exercise regularly is lower. At the same time, exercise can also reduce the possibility of fracture. Exercise can also improve body agility, strength, posture, balance, muscle strengthening, etc. It has the effect of reducing the risk of falling and reducing pain. Osteoporosis patients should pay more attention to improving tolerance and balance ability in the choice of exercise items. Here we recommend aerobic weight training or resistance exercises, such as walking, climbing stairs, jogging and Tai Chi, etc. The evidence shows that athletes in aerobic weight-bearing events have higher bone density than non-weight-bearing athletes such as bicycles and swimming.

2. 生活习惯管理

Lifestyle Management

纠正不良的生活习惯对避免或延缓骨质疏松症的发生也是相当重要的，戒烟限酒对骨质疏松症易患人群是有必要的。相较于其他疾病，骨质疏松症中比较需要注意的一个生活习惯是注意接收充足的日照，应尽可能多地暴露皮肤于阳光下晒15~30分钟，但需注意避免强烈的阳光所引起的皮肤灼伤。

Correcting bad living habits is also very important to avoid or delay the occurrence of osteoporosis. Quitting smoking and limiting alcohol is necessary for people who are susceptible to osteoporosis. Compared with other diseases, a life habit that needs attention in osteoporosis is to pay attention to receiving sufficient sunlight. Expose the skin to the sun as much as possible for 15-30 minutes. But take care to avoid skin burns caused by strong sunlight.

3. 相关监测管理

Related Monitoring

对于骨质疏松症患者或易感人群而言，比较重要的是对疾病的早期发现，也就是说尽早地发现骨密度的降低，及时进行干预，则完全可以避免后期骨折、全身性疼痛等症状的发生。

For patients with osteoporosis or susceptible people, it is more important to detect the disease early, that is, to detect the decrease in bone density as early as possible and to intervene in time can completely avoid the following occurrence of symptoms such as fractures, and generalized aches.

四、高尿酸血症患者的生活方式与健康管理

Section Four-Health Management of People with Hyperuricemia

（一）引言

Introduction

高尿酸血症是一种常见的代谢异常疾病之一。高尿酸血症形成的主要因素有两点，一者是尿酸盐生产过多，再者为肾脏尿酸排泄过少。随着我们生活水平的提高，我们的饮食结构已经发生了巨大的变化，更多的肉类、鱼类以及其他高嘌呤、高蛋白食物进入了我们的每日三餐中，人群尿酸水平逐渐升高，高尿酸血症的患病率也因此逐年上升。高尿酸血症并不是不可避免的，通过对高尿酸血症采取有效的健康管理，在很大程度上可以改善患者的生活质量，避免后续的并发症发生。

Hyperuricemia is one of the common metabolic disorders. There are two main causes of hyperuricemia. One is the excessive production of uric acid, and the other is the less excretion of uric acid by the kidneys. With the improvement of our living standards, our dietary structure has undergone tremendous changes. More meat, fish and other high-purine, high-protein foods have entered our three meals a day, and the uric acid level of the population has gradually increased, the prevalence of hyperuricemia has also increased year by year. However, hyperuricemia is evitable. Effective health management of hyperuricemia can improve the quality of life for patients to a large extent and avoid subsequent complications.

（二）高尿酸血症的形成

Causes of Hyperuricemia

当尿酸的产生过多或排泄减少时便可形成高尿酸血症。高尿酸血症的成因可分为三种类型，即尿酸生成增多、尿酸排泄减少以及二者混合型。

Hyperuricemia can be formed when the production of uric acid is too much or the excretion is reduced. The cause of hyperuricemia can be divided into three types, namely, increased uric acid production, decreased uric acid excretion, and a mixed type of the two.

（三）高尿酸血症的危害

Harm of Hyperuricemia

当各种原因引起循环尿酸含量升高超过血尿酸饱和浓度时，尿酸盐晶体会从血中析出，析出的尿酸盐结晶会在血液和组织中积累，从而引发炎症和组织损伤。高尿酸血症最常见的损害是痛风性的关节炎、关节痛风石形成、尿酸性尿石病以及慢性尿酸性肾病等。此外，有研究发现高尿酸血症与多种常见病存在着密切的联系，这包括了心血管疾病（高血压、冠心病等）、Ⅱ型糖尿病等。这可能与高尿酸水平下的炎症和激素吸收异常有关。

When the circulating uric acid content rises and exceeds the blood uric acid saturation concentration due to various reasons, urate crystals will be precipitated from the blood, and the precipitated urate crystals will accumulate in the blood and tissues, triggering inflammation and tissue damage. The most common damages are gouty arthritis, joint tophi, uric acid urolithiasis and chronic uric acid nephropathy. In addition, studies have found that hyperuricemia is closely related to a variety of common diseases, including cardiovascular diseases (hypertension, coronary heart disease, etc.), Type Ⅱ diabetes, etc. This may be related to the inflammation under high uric acid level and abnormal hormone absorption.

（四）高尿酸血症的健康管理

Health Management of Hyperuricemia

高尿酸血症已成为一种日趋常见的代谢性疾病，针对普通人群的干预主要通过提高大众对于该病症和痛风的认识，加强其健康管理的意识，进而降低人群发病率。健康管理也是高危人群必须要做的干预措施之一。应当了解疾病的发生机制，懂得如何进行高尿酸血症的预防。高尿酸血症的健康管理大致也包括运动管理、生活习惯管理、相关监测等方面。

Hyperuricemia has become an increasingly common metabolic disease. The intervention for the general population mainly aims to increase the public's awareness of the disease and gout, and strengthen their awareness of health management, thereby reducing the incidence of the population. Health management is also one of the intervention measures that high-risk groups must do. It is necessary to understand the mechanism of disease and how to prevent hyperuricemia. The health management of hyperuricemia also generally includes exercise management, lifestyle management, and related monitoring.

1. 运动管理

Exercise Management

规律、合理的运动可改善代谢，有效调节血尿酸水平，并减少痛风发作；但剧烈运动却可升高尿酸，诱发痛风，是痛风发作的第三位诱因。

Regular and reasonable exercise can improve metabolism, effectively regulate blood uric acid levels, and reduce gout attacks; but strenuous exercise can increase uric acid and induce gout, which is the third cause of gout attacks.

（1）合理运动

Exercise Moderately

高尿酸血症患者并非不能运动，而是合理运动。运动强度、运动时间是影响疾病转归的关键因素。应尽量避免高强度运动，如打篮球、踢足球等，高强度运动会消耗大量ATP，ATP代谢过程中会伴随尿酸生成，从而升高尿酸、诱发痛风。

Patients with hyperuricemia are not unable to exercise, but exercise reasonably. Exercise intensity and exercise time are the key factors affecting disease outcome. High-intensity exercises, such as playing basketball and football, should be avoided as much as possible. High-intensity exercise will consume a lot of ATP, and uric acid will be generated during ATP metabolism, which will increase uric acid and induce gout.

（2）体重控制

Weight Control

体重超重的患者，需要尽量减轻自己的体重，因为每减轻5千克，尿酸值也会相应地降低。

Overweight patients need to reduce their own weight as much as possible, because every 5 kilograms lost, the uric acid value will be correspondingly reduced.

2. 生活方式管理

Lifestyle Management

对于那些没有痛风症状并且没有心血管疾病或者代谢疾病的风险的患者，如果血尿酸较低，这类人群可以首先从生活方式上干预，一般经过3~6个月的生活干预后，再根据尿酸水平考虑进一步处理。具体干预方式应最好听从专业医生的指导。

For those who have no symptoms of gout and no risk of cardiovascular disease or metabolic disease, if their blood uric acid is lower, they may not use uric acid lowering drugs. Those people can intervene from the lifestyle first for 3-6 months, and then consider what to do according to the uric acid level. It is best to follow the guidance of a professional doctor.

（1）控制饮酒

Control Drinking

有研究发现啤酒的提高尿酸能力要强于酒精，因为啤酒中存在的嘌呤物质可以通过肠道细菌转为尿酸，葡萄酸对尿酸没有什么影响，所以高尿酸血症的患者最好不要喝白酒和啤酒，可以适量地喝红酒，但是不能喝太多。此外还需要注意有些含糖饮料也可以引发痛风的风险。

Studies have found that beer has a higher uric acid capacity than alcohol, because the presence of purine in beer can be converted to uric acid by intestinal bacteria. Gluconic acid has no effect on hyperuric acid, so it is best for patients with hyperuricemia not to drink white wine and beer. You can drink red wine in moderation, but not too much. In addition, it is worth noting that some sugary drinks can also cause the risk of gout.

（2）调节情绪

Regulate Emotion

有研究发现，人们在各种日常情绪压力下，血清中的尿酸水平会出现短暂升高，并会加重痛风发作的症状。尽管应激和尿酸之间的确切关系仍有待证明，但基于已有的结果，高尿酸血症患者应当合理调节情绪，避免应激。

Studies have found that under various daily emotional stresses, people's serum uric acid levels will temporarily increase, which will aggravate the symptoms of gout attacks. Although the exact relationship between stress and uric acid remains to be proved, based on the existing results, patients with hyperuricemia should adjust their emotions reasonably to avoid stress.

3. 相关监测

Related Monitoring

定期筛查血尿酸、尿酸检测，以保证可以早发现、早治疗。

Regular screening of blood uric acid and uric acid testing ensures early detection and early treatment.

五、血脂异常与脂蛋白异常血症患者的生活方式与健康管理

Section Five–Health Management of Dyslipidemia and Dyslipoproteinemia

（一）引言

Introduction

血脂异常是指血液中脂质含量异常，即脂质含量过多或脂质含量过少。随着我们生活水平的改善，如今绝大多数脂代谢异常者往往是高脂血症，即血脂升高，这往往是由我们不断丰富的饮食和静息的生活方式所造成的。本节所介绍的血脂异常指代的便是高脂血症。血脂异常所表现的脂质异常进一步引起了脂蛋白的异常，因此血脂异常可以表现为脂蛋白异常血症。

Dyslipidemia refers to the abnormal content of lipids in the blood, that is, hyperlipidemia or hypolipidemia. With the improvement of our living standards, the vast majority of people with abnormal lipid metabolism are often hyperlipidemia, that is, an elevation of lipids in the blood, which is often caused by our gradually enriching diet and resting lifestyle. The dyslipidemia described in this section refers to hyperlipidemia. Dyslipidemia further causes lipoprotein abnormalities, which can manifest as dyslipoproteinemia.

血脂异常与脂蛋白异常血症被认为是引起心脑血管疾病的主要危险因素之一。据世界卫生组织统计，每年大约有1700万人死于这种慢性疾病。此外，血脂异常还被认为增加了肿瘤的发生风险。因而，对血脂异常与脂蛋白异常血症进行合理的管理防治将极大地降低心血管疾病的患病率，对提高人群的生活质量具有重要的意义。

Dyslipidemia and dyslipoproteinemia are considered one of the major risk factors causing cardiovascular diseases. According to statistics from the World Health Organization, approximately 17 million people die from this chronic disease every year. In addition, dyslipidemia is also believed to increase the risk of tumors. Reasonable management and prevention of dyslipidemia and dyslipoproteinemia will greatly reduce the prevalence of cardiovascular diseases, and is of great significance to improve the quality of life of the population.

（二）血脂异常与脂蛋白异常血症的形成

Causes of Dyslipidemia and Dyslipoproteinemia

1. 血脂异常的类型与成因

Types and Causes of Dyslipidemia

当脂质代谢通路中的某一部分出现异常时，可出现脂质在血液中的聚集，导致高脂血症的形成。根据血脂异常的成因不同，分为原发性血脂异常与继发性血脂异常。

When a certain part of the lipid metabolism pathway is abnormal, lipids can accumulate in the blood, leading to the formation of hyperlipidemia. According to the different causes of dyslipidemia, dyslipidemia is clinically divided into two categories, namely primary dyslipidemia and secondary dyslipidemia.

（1）原发性血脂异常

Primary Dyslipidemia

原发性血脂异常占血脂异常的绝大多数，主要是由于遗传基因缺陷加之环境因素相互作用所引起的。由于是由遗传因素所引起的，所以原发性血脂异常往往呈现家族性聚集。在遗传缺陷的基础上，某些重要的环境因素如不良的饮食习惯、运动不足、肥胖、吸烟、过度饮酒等会加重血脂异常，从而形成高脂血症。

Primary dyslipidemia accounts for the vast majority of dyslipidemia, mainly due to genetic defects combined with the interaction of environmental factors. Gene defects can be manifested as single-gene defects or multi-gene defects, and different gene defects also manifest as different lipid component abnormalities. Because it is caused by genetic factors, primary dyslipidemia often presents familial aggregation. On the basis of genetic defects, certain important environmental factors such as poor eating habits, insufficient exercise, obesity, smoking, excessive drinking, etc. will aggravate dyslipidemia, thereby forming hyperlipidemia.

（2）继发性血脂异常

Secondary Dyslipidemia

继发性血脂异常是由另一种潜在疾病引起的，这种疾病会导致血脂和脂蛋白代谢的改变，这些疾病通过不同的机制影响了脂质运输。另外，某些药物也会引起脂质代谢的异常。

Secondary dyslipidemia is caused by another underlying disease, which can cause changes in blood lipids and lipoprotein metabolism. These diseases affect the lipid transport through different mechanisms. In addition, certain drugs can also cause abnormal lipid metabolism.

2. 原发性血脂异常的危险因素

Risk Factors of Primary Dyslipidemia

在血脂异常的成因中，我们提到了原发性血脂异常存在着环境因素的交互作用，这种环境因素即是血脂异常发生的危险因素。原发性血脂异常的危险因素可以分为可改变的危险因素与不可改变的危险因素。不可改变的危险因素主要包括了年龄、性别。一般而言男性的年龄达到45岁，女性的年龄达到55岁时，患上高脂血症的风险逐渐上升。可改变的危险因素包括了不健康的饮食、缺乏锻炼、吸烟等。身体缺乏足够的运动也往往会增加不良胆固醇的数量而减少有益的胆固醇。吸烟会损害血管壁，而血管壁的损伤会使得脂肪更容易聚集。

In the causes of dyslipidemia that we have mentioned above, primary dyslipidemia has an interaction of environmental factors. These environmental factors are risk factors for the occurrence of dyslipidemia. The risk factors of primary dyslipidemia can be divided into non-modifiable risk factors and modifiable risk factors. The non-modifiable risk factors mainly include age and gender. Generally speaking, when men reach 45 years old and women reach 55 years old, the risk of developing hyperlipidemia gradually increases. The risk factors that can be changed include unhealthy diet, lack of exercise, and smoking. Lack of enough exercise also tends to increase the number of bad cholesterol and reduce the good cholesterol. Smoking damages the blood vessel walls, and damage to the blood vessel walls makes it easier for fat to accumulate.

（三）血脂异常与脂蛋白异常血症的危害

Harm of Dyslipidemia and Dyslipoproteinemia

高脂血症最大的危害是其增加了动脉粥样硬化发生的可能性，高脂血症已被认为是发生动脉粥样硬化最重要的危险因素，而动脉粥样硬化是许多心脑血管疾病发病的主要成因。WHO最新资料显示，全球超过50%的冠心病的发生与胆固醇水平升高有关。动脉硬化也可以发生于脑血管中，可引起脑供血不足，增加了缺血性中风发生的风险。

The biggest danger of hyperlipidemia is that it increases the possibility of atherosclerosis. Hyperlipidemia has been recognized as the most important risk factor for atherosclerosis, and atherosclerosis is the main cause of many cardiovascular diseases. The latest survey from the WHO shows that more than 50% of the global coronary heart diseases are related to elevated cholesterol levels. Arteriosclerosis can also occur in cerebral vessels, which can cause insufficient blood supply to the brain and increase the risk of ischemic stroke.

（四）血脂异常与脂蛋白异常血症的健康管理

Health Management of Dyslipidemia and Dyslipoproteinemia

血脂异常健康管理的主要目标是控制血脂并预防动脉粥样硬化性所引起的相关心脑血管疾病，包括中风等。具体的不同脂质的异常可能需要不同的干预措施，这需要结合具体的管理策略。通常的健康管理策略包括了运动管理、生活方式管理。对于具有动脉硬化高危风险的人群，应尽早考虑进行调脂治疗，降低心脑血管事件的风险。

The main goal of dyslipidemia health management is to control blood lipids and prevent related cardiovascular and cerebrovascular diseases caused by atherosclerosis, including stroke, etc. The abnormality of a lipid may require different interventions, which need to be combined with specific management strategies. The usual health management strategies include exercise management, and lifestyle management. For people at high risk of arteriosclerosis, lipid-lowering therapy should be considered as early as possible to reduce the risk of cardiovascular and cerebrovascular events.

1. 运动管理

Exercise Management

血脂异常人群运动健身时应在运动处方的指导下科学地进行。选择合适的运动方式是获得良好锻炼效果的前提。能够改善身体机能的运动方式有许多种，如走跑锻炼、乒乓球、羽毛球、柔力球、游泳、骑自行车、跳交谊舞、跳绳、太极拳、秧歌、登山、力量练习等，但它们并不都能使血脂异常得到有效改善。其中，走跑锻炼是治疗血脂异常的一种有效的运动，可作为首选的调脂运动方式。走跑锻炼的形式包括走或跑，其动作要求为抬头挺胸收腹、双眼平视、肩部放松、肘部弯曲约90度，并随走跑节奏前后摆动手臂。

People with dyslipidemia should exercise scientifically under the guidance of exercise prescriptions. The choice of exercise mode is the prerequisite for good exercise effect. There are many types of exercises that can improve physical function, such as walking and running, table tennis, badminton, soft ball, swimming, cycling, ballroom dancing, rope skipping, Tai Chi, Yangko, mountaineering, strength exercises, etc., but not all of them can effectively improve dyslipidemia. Among them, walking and running exercise is an effective exercise to treat dyslipidemia, and can be adopted as the first choice for lipid-lowering exercise. The form of walking and running exercise includes walking or running. The action requirements are to raise your head, chest and abdomen, look straight, relax your shoulders, bend your elbows about 90 degrees, and swing arms back and forth with the rhythm of walking.

进行走跑锻炼时，运动强度不是影响血脂异常改善效果的主要因素，低强度的走跑锻炼就可收到较好的改善血脂异常的作用，而中等强度的走跑锻炼并不能带来更多的有益性改变。每次锻炼的持续时间比运动强度更为重要，较为全面的血脂状况改善要在较长的锻炼周期（6个月）后才能出现。因此，锻炼要持之以恒。根据研究，走跑锻炼的运动强度为最大心率的

50%~60%。

During walking and running exercise, exercise intensity is not the main factor that affects the effect of improving dyslipidemia. Low-intensity walking and running exercises can have a better effect on improving dyslipidemia, while moderate-intensity walking and running exercises cannot bring more beneficial changes. The duration of each exercise is more important than the intensity of the exercise. A more comprehensive improvement in blood lipid status can only appear after a longer exercise cycle (6 months). Therefore, one should do exercise persistently. According to research, the exercise intensity of walking and running exercise is 50% to 60% of the maximum heart rate.

2. 生活方式管理

Lifestyle Management

吸烟是导致心血管疾病发病率高的重要原因，应完全戒烟和避免吸入二手烟，这能很好地预防心血管疾病。可通过健康教育，专门的戒烟门诊、戒烟热线以及药物的辅助来帮助抽烟的血脂异常人群成功戒烟。

Smoking is an important reason for the high incidence of cardiovascular disease. You should completely quit smoking and avoid inhaling second-hand smoke, which can prevent cardiovascular disease. Health education, special smoking cessation clinics, smoking cessation hotlines, and drug assistance can help smokers with dyslipidemia successfully quit smoking.

低中危动脉粥样硬化性心血管疾病风险者，在启动降脂药物治疗前，需要先进行至少3个月的生活方式干预后再重新评估是否需要药物治疗；而高危动脉粥样硬化性心血管疾病风险者，生活方式干预和药物治疗需同时进行。

People with low and medium-risk atherosclerotic cardiovascular disease risk need to undergo lifestyle intervention for at least 3 months before starting lipid-lowering drug therapy and reassessing whether they need drug treatment; while for people at high-risk of atherosclerotic heart disease, lifestyle intervention and drug treatment must be carried out at the same time.

第二节 运动方式与健康管理
Section Two Exercise Mode and Health Management

运动损伤是在运动过程中发生的各类损伤，在临床上非常常见，常常是由于人们缺乏运动常识和安全意识造成的。运动损伤会给人们带来极坏的生理和心理影响，妨碍体育锻炼的正常进行。运动损伤应该遵循"以防为主、防治结合"的原则，在深入研究运动损伤产生的原因、机理和规律的基础上，针对性地制定防治措施，加强对体育锻炼安全的宣传，有利于降低运动损伤发生率及其危害程度。

Sports injuries are all kinds of injuries that occur during exercise, which are very common in clinical practice, and it is often caused by people's lack of sports knowledge and safety awareness. Treatment of sports injuries can bring extremely bad physical and psychological effects to people and hinder the normal progress of exercise. Sports injuries should follow the principle of "prevention and treatment, mainly in prevention", based on in-depth research on the causes, mechanisms and laws of sports injuries. Targeted prevention and treatment measures should be formulated, and the promotion of safety in physical exercise should be strengthened, which is beneficial to reduce the incidence of sports injuries and the degree of harm.

一、有关预防常见运动损伤的理论知识

Section One-Knowledge about Preventing Common Sports Injuries

（一）运动损伤的定义

Definition of Sports Injuries

运动损伤指在运动过程中所发生的各种损伤，它是运动医学的重要组成部分，其主要任务是预防和治疗运动中的损伤，研究运动损伤的发生原因、发病规律、预防措施、现场急救处理及治疗措施等。常见的运动损伤主要包括：开放性软组织损伤、闭合性软组织损伤、腹腔内部的运动创伤、脊柱骨折及脑震荡等。其损伤部位与运动项目以及专项技术特点有关，如体操运动员受伤部位多是腕、肩及腰部，与体操动作中的支撑、转肩、跳跃、翻腾等技术有关。网球肘多发生于网球运动员与标枪运动员。

Sports injury refers to various injuries that occur during exercise. It is an important part of sports medicine. Its main task is to prevent and treat injuries in sports, study the causes of sports injuries, the law of onset, preventive measures, first aid on site and treatment measures, etc. Common sports injuries mainly include: open soft tissue injuries, closed soft tissue injuries, sports injuries in the abdominal cavity, spinal fractures and concussions. The injury parts are related to sports events and special techniques. For example, the injured parts of gymnasts are mostly wrists, shoulders and waists, which are related to the support, shoulder turning, jumping, and tossing in gymnastics. Tennis elbow occurs mostly in tennis players and javelin throwers.

（二）几种常见运动损伤的定义及其处理建议

Definitions and Treatment Suggestions of Several Common Sports Injuries

1. 重力性休克

Gravitational Shock

（1）定义

Definition

重力性休克是一种暂时性的血管调节发生障碍所引起的急性脑缺血，会导致全身软弱、头晕、恶心、呕吐、出冷汗、脸色苍白、脉搏跳动缓慢而弱、呼吸缓慢、甚至晕倒的现象。主要是由于参加赛跑（特别是短、中距离）到达终点后，突然停下来，站立不动，此时下肢扩张的毛细血管和静脉失去了肌肉收缩对它们的挤压而产生的"肌肉泵"作用，血液因受重力的影响，大量的血液积聚在下肢血管中，这导致上腔静脉回流困难，回心血量和心输出量减少，使脑部的血液供应暂时减少而发生的急性脑贫血。

Gravitational shock is an acute cerebral ischemia caused by a temporary disorder of vascular regulation, which leads to body weakness, dizziness, nausea, vomiting, cold sweats, pale face, slow and weak pulse, slow breathing, and even fainting phenomenon. It mostly takes place after participating in the race (especially the short and middle distances) to the end, when people suddenly stop and stand still. At this time, the expanded capillaries and veins of the lower limbs lose the "muscle pump" that is squeezed by their muscles. Due to the influence of gravity, a large amount of blood accumulates in the blood vessels of the lower extremities, which makes the superior vena cava difficult to return. The return to the heart blood volume and cardiac output are reduced, and the blood supply to the brain is temporarily reduced and the acute cerebral anemia occurs.

（2）处理建议

Treatment Suggestions

对于身体健康的人出现这种现象并不危险，应让休克者仰卧，两腿抬起高于头（保持静脉血回流到心脏），松开衣领、腰带、注意保暖，不省人事时可掐人中穴，清醒后喝点热水或热糖水，充分静卧、保暖和休息。

This phenomenon is not dangerous for people who are in good health. People in shock should lie on their back, raise their legs above their heads (to keep venous blood flowing back to the heart), loosen the collar and belt, and keep warm.

2. 脑震荡

Concussion

（1）定义

Definition

脑震荡是指头部受到外力打击或碰撞后，脑功能发生暂时性障碍。在运动损伤中，脑震荡较多发生在足球、摩托车、拳击、投掷、体操等运动过程中。脑震荡发生时，受伤者会立即出现神志昏迷，意志丧失，一般在数分钟到半小时后方才清醒，脉搏、呼吸微弱，并伴有不同程度的头昏、头痛、恶心、呕吐等症状。

Concussion refers to the temporary impairment of brain function after the head is hit or hit by an external force. Among sports injuries, concussions often occur during sports such as football, motorcycles, boxing, throwing, and gymnastics. When a concussion occurs, the injured people will immediately become unconscious. Generally, they will wake up after a few minutes to half an hour, with weak pulse and breathing, and varying degrees of dizziness, headache, nausea, and vomiting.

（2）处理建议

Treatment Suggestions

脑震荡发生后，应立即让伤者平卧，绝对保持安静。严禁摇动、牵扯，更不要随意移动位置，头部两侧用衣物填塞，以免左右摇晃，同时用毛巾浸湿冷敷头部，身体衣着要保暖。病情严重者应立即送医院抢救。

After a concussion, the injured person should be placed on his back and absolutely kept quiet. It is strictly forbidden to shake, pull, or move the position randomly. Fill the sides of the head with clothing to avoid shaking left and right. At the same time, use a towel to soak the head and keep warm.

3. 关节脱位

Joint Dislocation

（1）定义

Definition

在外力作用下，使关节面彼此失去正常的连接关系，称为关节脱位，又叫脱臼。关节脱位一般都会引起关节囊撕裂和关节周围的韧带肌腱及其附着组织的损伤。

Under the action of external force, the articular surfaces lose their normal connection relationship with each other, which is called joint dislocation. Joint dislocation generally causes tearing of the joint capsule and damage to the ligaments, tendons and attached tissues around the joints.

第八章 生活方式与健康管理
CHAPTER EIGHT LIFE STYLE AND HEALTH MANAGEMENT

（2）处理建议

Treatment Suggestions

关节脱位后，应首先进行止痛抗休克，然后固定脱位关节，不得使之移动，更不能随意使用整复手法，应迅速护送到医院进行整复、治疗。

After joint dislocation, you should first perform pain relief and anti-shock, and then fix the dislocated joint without moving it, let alone using rehabilitation techniques at will. You should quickly escort the injured to the hospital for rehabilitation and treatment.

4. 骨折

Fracture

（1）定义

Definition

骨折是指由于外力的作用，骨的完整性和连接性遭到了破坏。骨折分为闭合性骨折和开放性骨折。

Fracture refers to the destruction of bone integrity and connectivity due to external forces. Fractures are divided into closed fractures and open fractures.

（2）症状

Symptoms

①疼痛

Pain

刚发生骨折时，疼痛较轻，但随后因周围软组织和骨膜撕裂、肌肉痉挛等，疼痛感变得剧烈，严重的可使人发生休克。

When a fracture occurs, the pain is mild. But then the pain becomes severe due to tearing of the surrounding soft tissues and periostea, muscle spasms, etc. What's worse, it way cause a state of shock.

②肿胀和皮下淤血

Swelling and Congestion Under the Skin

骨折后因疼痛、肌肉痉挛，由于骨骼工作失去的原有的杠杆作用及软组织的损害，伤者多不能站立、行走或活动，骨折部位畸形、异常活动和伴有骨擦声，有压痛和震痛感，可用X光片检查证实。

After the fracture, due to pain, muscle spasm, loss of original leverage and soft tissue damage due to skeletal work, most of the injured cannot stand, walk or move. The fracture site is deformed, abnormal moved and accompanied by bone rubbing, and there is tenderness and tremor. It can be confirmed by X-ray examination.

（3）处理建议

Treatment Suggestions

骨折发生后，切不可随意复位，以免加重损伤，应当安全护送到医院。

After the fracture, do not reset it at will in case of aggravating the injury. The injured should be safely escorted to the hospital.

5. 疲劳性骨膜炎

Fatigue Periostitis

（1）定义

Definition

由于肌肉不断收缩，牵拉骨膜，骨膜松弛出血，引起骨膜炎。胫腓骨是常发生疲劳性骨膜炎的部位，特别是冬季长跑，常由于足尖跑跳多、马路较硬、腿部力量不足等原因所致。

As the muscles continue to contract and stretch the periosteum, the periosteum relaxes and bleeds, causing periostitis. Tibia and fibula is the site of fatigue periostitis, especially in winter long-distance running. It is often caused by too much toes running and jumping, the hard road, and the insufficient leg strength.

（2）症状

Symptoms

跑步时，后蹬疼痛是胫腓骨骨膜炎的特殊征象，局部出血，皮肤发红发热，有时局部水肿；有明显压痛，压痛区内能摸到骨面小结节。

When running, kicking pain is a special sign of tibiofibular periostitis, with local bleeding, skin redness and heat, and sometimes local edema. There is obvious tenderness, and small nodules on the bone surface can be felt in the tender area.

（3）处理建议

Treatment Suggestions

患胫腓骨骨膜炎时，应同时包裹弹力绷带，进行按摩、理疗；减少跑量或停止长跑，局部封闭。

When suffering from tibia and fibula periostitis, elastic bandages should be wrapped at the same time, with massage and physical therapy. Reduce the amount of running or stop long-distance running with local blocking.

6. 膝盖损伤

Knee Injury

（1）定义

Definition

膝关节是全身最大的屈伸关节，主要做屈伸运动，因其位于下肢的中部，位于身体两个最大的杠杆臂之间，承受较大的力，易引起扭伤和骨折。膝盖损伤指由于外界的碰撞或长期劳损、过度疲劳而导致的膝关节软组织及骨或软骨的损伤。在体育活动中膝关节的韧带及半月板损伤极为常见。

The knee joint is the largest flexor joint in the whole body. It is mainly used for flexion and extension. It bears great force and is easy to suffer from sprains and fractures because it is located in the middle of the lower limbs, which are the two largest lever arms of the body. Knee injury refers to the damage to the soft tissues and bones or cartilages of the knee joint due to external collisions, long-term strain, and excessive fatigue. In sports activities, knee ligaments and half-month injuries are extremely common.

（2）症状

Symptoms

急性期主要表现为关节肿胀、疼痛、关节积液及屈伸活动受限；急性期过后疼痛感降低，但在进行上下楼梯等膝盖负重的活动时疼痛感明显。膝盖损伤一般占所有运动损伤的55%，涉及的运动包括跑步、自行车、游泳、足球、篮球、排球等。

The acute stage is mainly manifested as joint swelling, pain, joint effusion, and limited flexion and extension activities. After the acute stage, the pain is reduced, but the pain is obvious when performing knee weight-bearing activities such as going up and downstairs. Knee injuries generally account for 55% of all sports injuries. Running, cycling, swimming, football, basketball, volleyball and other sports are involved.

（3）处理建议

Treatment Suggestions

膝盖损伤急性期应进行休息，避免膝关节剧烈运动。进行相关运动时建议应常更换运动鞋及鞋垫；运动场地要软一点；多进行锻炼四头肌的力量练习。

In the acute stage of knee injury, rest should be carried out to avoid severe exercise of knee joint. It is suggested that sports shoes and insoles should be replaced frequently when carrying out relevant exercises; the sports field should be soft; more exercise on quadriceps strength should be done.

7. 肩伤

Shoulder Injury

（1）定义

Definition

肩伤指因肩部各组织包括肩袖、韧带发生退行性改变，或因反复过度使用、创伤等原因造成的肩关节周围组织的损伤。约20%的运动损伤会涉及到肩部，比如错位、扭伤和拉伤等。肩伤在网球、游泳、举重、棒球和排球中最常见。

Shoulder injury refers to the degenerative changes of shoulder tissues including rotator cuff and ligament, or the injury of tissues around the shoulder joint caused by repeated overuse and trauma. About 20% of sports injuries involve the shoulder injury, such as dislocation, sprain and strain. Shoulder injuries are most common in tennis, swimming, weightlifting, baseball and volleyball.

（2）症状

Symptoms

主要症状有疼痛、僵硬、无力等。

The main symptoms are pain, stiffness and weakness.

（3）处理建议

Treatment Suggestions

受伤后，先冷敷受伤部位，再压迫及抬高受伤部位；建议平时应多活动肩部。

After the injury, you can apply cold compress to the injured part first, then press and raise the injured part. It is suggested to move the shoulder more often.

8.踝关节扭伤

Ankle Sprain

（1）定义

Definition

踝关节扭伤常常是因为踝关节周围的韧带损伤导致的，相关的韧带主要有3组：内侧副韧带、外侧副韧带和下胫腓韧带。根据损伤韧带的不同，踝关节扭伤可以分为3类：内侧踝关节扭伤、外侧踝关节扭伤和高位踝关节扭伤。

Ankle sprain is often caused by ligament damage around the ankle joint. The related ligaments are mainly medial collateral ligament, lateral collateral ligament and inferior tibiofibular ligament. According to the different ligaments, ankle sprains can be divided into three types: medial ankle sprains, lateral ankle sprains and high ankle sprains.

（2）症状

Symptoms

肿胀、疼痛及行走障碍等。踝关节外翻扭伤虽不易发生，一旦出现却很严重。如发生断裂，一般都会引起踝关节不稳，并且很多时候会同时伴有其他韧带损伤和骨折。踝关节扭伤约占所有运动损伤的40%。脚踝扭伤在足球、曲棍球、篮球和排球运动中最为常见，在跑、跳及快速转动运动中几乎难以避免。

Swelling, pain and walking disorders. Although ankle valgus sprain is not easy to occur, once it occurs, it is very serious. If fracture occurs, it will generally cause ankle instability, and often accompanied by other ligament injuries and fractures. Ankle sprain accounts for about 40% of all sports injuries. Ankle sprain is the most common in football, hockey, basketball and volleyball. It is almost unavoidable in running, jumping and fast rotation.

（3）处理建议

Treatment Suggestions

如果发生踝关节扭伤，按照RICE原则进行处理，然后尽快送医。就诊后由医生对伤情进行评估，并决定治疗方案。

If ankle sprain occurs, the injured should be treated according to RICE principle, and then sent to the doctor as soon as possible. After treatment, the doctor evaluates the injury and decides the treatment plan.

9. 肌肉拉伤

Muscle Strain

（1）定义

Definition

肌肉拉伤是肌肉在运动中急剧收缩或过度牵拉引起的损伤，所以在完成引体向上和仰卧起坐等需要肌肉牵拉的项目时，如果动作不到位，非常容易发生。

Muscle strain is a kind of injury caused by rapid contraction or excessive stretching of muscles in sports, so it is very easy to occur if the action is not correct when completing pull-up and sit ups and other sports that need muscle traction.

（2）症状
Symptoms

如果拉伤部位剧痛，用手可摸到肌肉紧张形成的索条状硬块，触疼明显，局部肿胀或皮下出血，肢体活动明显受到限制，则可大致断定为肌肉拉伤。也可以通过肌肉抗阻力试验，简便地检测。其做法是：患者做受伤肌肉的主动收缩活动，检查者对该活动施加一定阻力，在对抗过程中出现疼痛的部位，即为拉伤肌肉的损伤处。

If there is a sharp pain in the injured part, a cable like hard mass formed by muscle tension that can be felt by hand, with obvious touch pain, local swelling or subcutaneous bleeding, and obvious limitation of limb movement, then it can be roughly determined as muscle strain. It can also be easily detected by muscle resistance test. The method is: the patient takes the active contraction activity of the injured muscle, and the examiner applies certain resistance to the activity. The part with pain in the process of confrontation is the injured part of the pulled muscle.

（3）处理建议
Treatment Suggestions

确认肌肉拉伤后，要立即进行冷敷，用冷水冲局部或用毛巾包裹冰决冷敷，然后用绷带适当用力包裹损伤部位，防止肿胀。24小时至48小时后拆除包扎，可外贴活血贴，消除肿胀，也可适当热敷或用较轻的手法对损伤局部进行按摩。

After confirming the muscle strain, immediately apply cold compress, wash the part with cold water or wrap it with towel, and then wrap the injured part with bandage to prevent swelling. After 24 hours to 48 hours, remove the bandage and apply plaster to eliminate the swelling. You can also apply hot compress or massage the injured area with a lighter stimulus.

10. 运动性腹痛
Exercise Induced Abdominal Pain

（1）定义

Definition

运动中腹痛是由激烈运动引起的一时性的机能紊乱，这并不是疾病，随着运动停止，症状可以逐渐缓解。运动性腹痛的成因大致有四种，分别是胃肠痉挛、肝脾区疼痛、腹直肌痉挛和腹部慢性疾病。

Abdominal pain during exercise is a temporary functional disorder caused by intense exercise, which is not a disease. With the cessation of exercise, the symptoms can be gradually relieved. There are four causes of exercise-induced abdominal pain: gastrointestinal spasm, liver and spleen pain, rectus abdominis spasm and chronic abdominal diseases.

（2）症状

Symptoms

运动性腹痛除腹痛外一般不伴随其他症状，经常安静时不痛，运动时才痛；疼痛程度与运动量强度成正比。

In addition to abdominal pain, exercise-induced abdominal pain is generally not accompanied by other symptoms, most of which are not painful at rest, but painful only during exercise. The degree of pain is directly proportional to the intensity of exercise.

（3）处理建议

Treatment Suggestions

如果还没有对腹痛明确诊断，不能随意服用止痛药，防止掩盖病情造成误诊。一般运动过程中腹痛时，可适当减速，调整呼吸，并以手按压。如果上述方法运用后，疼痛仍不减轻并有所加重时，应立即停止运动。如仍不见效，送医院诊治，以排除腹腔内或腹腔外疾病。

If there is no clear diagnosis of abdominal pain, we cannot take painkillers at will in case of misdiagnosis. If the pain is not relieved and aggravated after using the above methods, stop the exercise immediately. If it is still ineffective, send the patient to the hospital for diagnosis and treatment, so as to exclude intra-abdominal or extra-abdominal diseases.

11. 运动碰撞导致的鼻流血

Nosebleed Caused by Sports Collision

（1）定义

Definition

鼻出血是鼻子受外部力量的撞击后鼻腔毛细血管破裂所致，在激烈对抗活动中很容易发生。

Nosebleed is caused by the rupture of nasal capillaries after the nose is impacted by external forces. It is easy to happen in the fierce confrontation.

（2）症状

Symptoms

如果在碰撞后鼻梁骨疼痛，并且流血，有可能是软组织损伤，以及鼻梁骨骨折。

If the nasal bone is painful and bleeding after the collision, it may be soft tissue injury and fracture of the nasal bone.

（3）处理建议

Treatment Suggestions

如果疼痛不是很严重，并且血止住了就不用太过在意，用冰袋冷敷，止血，预防血肿就可以。如果很痛，则有可能鼻梁骨骨折，需要到医院拍片确诊，防止更严重的伤病。

If the pain is not very serious, and the blood stopped, you don't have to care too much, and you can use an ice bag to cold compress, stop bleeding, and prevent hematoma. If it is very painful, it may be nasal bone fracture, which needs you to go to the hospital to take film diagnosis, to prevent more serious injuries.

（二）运动损伤的分类

Classification of Sports Injuries

区分不同的运动损伤类型，有利于患者在运动损伤发生之后能够快速找到行之有效的解决方案，以免因用错方法或错过最佳处理时间导致更严重的后果。运动损伤可进行四个维度的分类：

Distinguishing different types of sports injury is helpful for patients to quickly find effective solutions after sports injury, so as to avoid more serious consequences caused by using the wrong method or missing the best treatment time. Sports injury can be classified into four dimensions:

按照伤后皮肤是否完整，可以分为开放性损伤和闭合性损伤。

According to whether the skin is intact after injury, it can be divided into open injury and closed injury.

按照伤后病程的阶段，可分为急性损伤、慢性损伤。

According to the stage of post injury course, it can be divided into acute injury and chronic injury.

按照受伤的组织结构，可以分为肌肉损伤、肌腱损伤、四肢骨折、内脏损伤等。

According to the tissue structure of the injury, it can be divided into muscle injury, tendon injury, limb fracture, visceral injury, etc.

按照损伤的轻重程度，可分为轻伤、中等伤、重伤。

According to the severity of the injury, it can be divided into mild injury, moderate injury and serious injury.

（三）运动损伤的成因

Causes of Sports Injuries

1. 缺乏预防运动损伤的知识，预防意识不强

Lack of Knowledge of Strong Sports Injury Prevention

运动损伤作为运动过程中发生的各种损伤，普遍发生在生活中每一个角落，大多是因为人们缺乏预防运动损伤的基本知识，或者没有意识到预防运动损伤的重要性，比如在训练前的准备活动不充分、不合理，教练员忽视了训练过程中适当放松的必要性等。

Sports injury, as a variety of injuries in the process of sports, generally occurs in every corner of life, mostly because people lack the basic knowledge of preventing sports injury, or they do not realize the importance of preventing sports injury, such as inadequate and unreasonable preparation activities before training, coaches' ignoring the necessity of appropriate relaxation in the process of training, etc.

2. 缺乏准备活动或准备活动不科学

Lack of Preparation or Unscientific Preparation

相当一部分普通锻炼者在正式开始锻炼前，不做准备活动或准备活动不充分，这会增加运动损伤发生的概率。

A considerable number of ordinary exercisers do not do preparatory activities or do not do enough preparatory activities before they begin to exercise, which will increase the probability of sports injury.

准备活动的内容与运动的基本内容结合不好，缺乏有针对性的专门性准备活动，运动中负担较重部位的机能没有改善，容易使特定部位受伤。

The content of preparatory activities is not well combined with the basic content of sports and lack of targeted and specialized preparatory activities, and the function of the parts with heavy burden in sports is not improved, so it is easy to make the specific parts injured.

准备活动运动量过大，会使身体提前进入疲劳状态，当进入正式运动时，身体机能下降，在这种情况下容易引起运动损伤。

The excessive amount of preparatory exercise will make the body enter the fatigue state ahead of time. When entering the formal exercise, the body function declines; in this case, it is easy to cause sports injury.

3. 运动内容和强度选择的不科学

Unscientific Sports Activities and Intensity

（1）运动内容不科学

Unscientific Sports Activities

在训练过程中，教练员忽视了训练过程中适当放松的必要性，安排了与受训者体能水平不相符的运动内容，或者是一些运动员为了提高自己的比赛成绩和竞技技术坚持带伤训练，以及教练未组织好训练项目，尤其是具有对抗性的训练项目。运动员的生理因素一定程度上对运动能力有所限制，若运动员和教练员未意识到这一点，安排与自己生理水平不符的训练项目，极容易造成运动损伤。

In the process of training, coaches ignore the need to relax properly in the process of training and arrange sports activities which is not consistent with the level of physical fitness of the trainees. Some athletes insist on training with injuries in order to improve their competition performance and competitive skills, and the coaches do not organize the training items well, especially the antagonistic training items. To some extent, athletes' physiological factors limit their sports ability. If athletes and coaches do not realize this and arrange training items that are not in line with their own physiological level, it is very easy to cause sports injuries.

（2）运动强度不合理

Unreasonable Sports Intensity

运动负荷（尤其是局部负担量）安排过大，没有充分考虑到锻炼者的生理特点，运动负荷超过了锻炼者可以承受的生理负担量，尤其是局部负担过大，引起微细损伤的积累而发生劳损，这是体育专项训练中造成运动损伤的主要原因。这里需要指出的是，疲劳并不等于运动过量，运动本身就是产生疲劳的项目，它通过产生疲劳—消除疲劳这个过程，使人体得到锻炼，加强肌肉力量和各器官的协调，减缓身体随年龄老化的程度。疲劳是身体的自然反应，如果出汗、腰膝酸软、肌肉疼痛等一些急性疲劳现象在下次运动时能够恢复，就不算是运动过量。相反，才被称为运动过量。

When the exercise load (especially the local load) is too large, the physiological characteristics of the exerciser are not fully considered and the exercise load exceeds the physiological load that the exerciser can bear, especially the local load is too large, which causes the accumulation of micro injury and strain that is the main cause of sports injury in sports special training. It should be pointed out here that fatigue is not equal to excessive exercise. Exercise itself is an item that produces fatigue. It exercises the human body through the process of producing fatigue and recovering fatigue, strengthens the coordination of muscle strength and various organs, and slows down the aging process of the body. Fatigue is a natural reaction of the body. If sweating, waist and knee soreness, muscle pain and other acute fatigue phenomenon can recover before the next exercise, the exercise is not excessire. The contrary is called excessive exercise.

（3）运动项目选择较单一

Single Choice of Sports

进行过于单一的运动项目也容易运动过量，造成过度疲劳。如在跑步项目中运动员极容易发生踝关节扭伤，跟腱拉伤，此外长跑还会造成疲劳性骨膜炎。跳跃项目则容易产生足跟挫伤、腰肌扭伤。投掷项目会损伤运动员的肩部、肘部、膝部的关节与肌肉。因此，应该选择多样化的运动方式，培养多元化的运动乐趣。每周进行不同的运动项目，既全方位锻炼了身体，也避免了单一运动造成的劳损。

Doing a single sport too much can also be prone to excessive exercise, resulting in excessive fatigue. For example, in running events, athletes are prone to ankle sprain, achilles tendon strain. In addition, long-distance running will cause fatigue periostitis. Jumping is easy to produce heel contusion and lumbar muscle sprain. Throwing events will damage the shoulder, elbow, knee joints and muscles of athletes. Therefore, we should choose a variety of sports and cultivate a variety of sports fun. Doing different sports every week, can not only achieve all-round exercise, but also avoid the strain caused by a single exercise.

从专业角度来说，运动过量会产生两种后果，一种是竞技体育的过度训练，另一个就是普通运动的过度疲劳。这种疲劳一般是慢性的，通过每一次没有完全恢复的运动疲劳的积累，导致人体出现种种不适症状。常见的膝关节劳损、腰背肌慢性劳损，就是局部过度疲劳的后果。而这种情况下就需要改变锻炼方式，比如经常打篮球的人应该减少打球次数，穿插其他运动来代替单一的运动。当你在运动后出现反应能力下降、平衡感降低、肌肉的弹性减小，一到运动场地就出现头晕恶心、抑郁、易怒等状态时，这很有可能是整体过度疲劳造成的神经官能症，应立即停止运动就医。为了避免运动过量等带来过度疲劳，人们在运动时要循序渐进、因人而异，根据个人年龄和身体状况选择运动项目和安排运动强度。

From a professional point of view, excessive exercise will produce two consequences, one is the overtraining of competitive sports, the other is the overtraining of ordinary sports. This kind of fatigue is generally chronic, which is formed through the accumulation of exercise fatigue that has not been fully recovered every time, and it leads to a variety of discomfort symptoms in the human body. Common knee joint strain and chronic strain of lumbodorsal muscle are the result of local fatigue. And in this case, we need to change the way of exercise. For example, people who often play basketball should reduce the frequenly and be interspersed with other sports instead of doing a single sport. When you have decreased reaction ability, decreased sense of balance, decreased elasticity of muscles, dizziness, nausea, depression and irritability, it is very likely that fatigue causes neurosis. You should stop exercising immediately and seek medical advice. In order to avoid excessive fatigue caused by excessive exercise, people should choose sports and arrange exercise intensity according to their age and physical condition.

4. 运动技术水平要求过高

High Requirement of Sports Skill Level

人们选择的运动内容具有一定的复杂性，而往往大多数人缺乏一定的技术水平。

The choice of sports activities has a certain degree of complexity, but most people often lack a certain level of technology.

一些人对高难度的技术动作理解不到位就进行错误操作，违背了人体运动的生物力学原理从而产生运动损伤。

If the individual's understanding of difficult technical movements is not enough, the wrong operation is carried out, which violates the biomechanical principle of human movement, resulting in sports injury.

技术动作操作不熟练。由于体育运动训练对训练者的反应力有着较高的要求，假若训练者对于技术动作操作不熟悉，意识没有跟上身体动作，就会导致损伤的发生。

Unskilled technical operation. Due to higher requirements of the trainers' reaction ability in sports training, if the trainers are not familiar with the operation of technical movements and their consciousness does not keep up with the body movements, the injury will occur.

5. 身体机能和心理状态不良

Poor Physical and Mental Functioning

因身体、心理状态不良而发生的运动损伤往往多发于青少年。青少年生理发育正处于青春期末期，身体机能基本上成熟，但是心理状态往往呈现出较为冲动、争强好胜的特点，尤其体育运动本来带有竞技性特征，训练中会存在受训者为了满足虚荣心而忽视自己的实际水平做出一些高难度动作的现象。心理上的不成熟还表现在无法较好地控制自身的情绪，使得情绪对运动员本身行为产生较大影响。生理因素主要包括肌肉力量、柔韧性、灵敏度、协调性、损伤史、疲劳程度。其中造成运动损伤最主要的原因为肌肉力量不足、柔韧性不足以及身体处于过度疲劳状态。

Physical and psychological sports injuries due to poor state often occur in teenagers. Teenagers' physical development is at the end of puberty, and their physical functions are basically mature, but their psychological state often presents the characteristics of impulsive and competitive, coupled with the competitive characteristics of sports. In training, there will be some difficult movements that trainees done because they ignore their actual level in order to satisfy their vanity.

Psychological immaturity is also reflected in the inability to better control their own emotions which have a greater impact on the athletes' own behavior. Physiological factors include muscle strength, flexibility, sensitivity, coordination, injury history and fatigue degree. Among them, the main causes of sports injury are lack of muscle strength, lack of flexibility and body fatigue.

6. 项目的特殊性（对抗性运动易造成损伤）

Particularity in Discipline (Competitive Sports are Easy to Cause Injuries)

有些体育运动为了一定的观赏性，对运动员的肢体活动有所要求。篮球、足球等需要与人面对面竞技，需要较强的身体对抗。在这种类型的体育运动中很容易发生肢体碰撞从而造成运动损伤。球类运动中，篮球对运动员的身体素质要求最高，在运动过程中具有较为强烈的对抗性，因此很容易发生指关节挫伤、韧带拉伤、腰部扭伤等，如著名篮球运动员姚明，在与快船队的比赛中，与蒂姆·托马斯相撞，导致右膝盖胫骨骨裂，因此被迫休息了32场比赛。足球与篮球一样，对抗过程中较多的奔跑与争抢容易产生巨大的身体冲突，较强的外部冲击力容易导致擦伤或骨折等运动损伤。

Some sports need athletes' physical activities in order to get a certain degree of visual enjoyment. Sports such as basketball and football need face-to-face competition and strong physical confrontation. In this type of sports, it is very easy to have body collision, which will cause sports injury. In ball games, basketball has the highest requirements on the physical quality of athletes, and has a strong antagonism in the process of deing sports, so it is easy to lead to finger joint contusion, ligament strain, waist sprain, etc. For example, the famous basketball player Yao Ming, in the game with the Clippers, collided with Tim Thomas, resulting in right knee tibial fracture, so he was forced to rest for 32 games. Football, like basketball, is easy to cause many physical conflicts in the process of running and fighting. Strong external impact force is easy to cause sports injuries such as bruises or fractures.

7. 场地、设备、服装上的缺陷

Defects in Site, Equipment and Clothing

场地不平整，器械的大小、重量与年龄、性别不相适应，着装不符合要求等，都是引起损伤的重要原因。

Uneven site, the size and weight of the equipment that do not match the age and gender, and that the clothing does not meet the requirements are the important reasons for the injury.

此外，练习场地声音、录像等设备不足或过多而影响听觉、视觉，会使大脑做出错误的判断；光线不足或过量，会使神经反应迟钝或过快，这些都有可能造成运动损伤。因此，为避免损伤的发生，练前要仔细检查器材是否安全，加强思想安全教育，遵守各项安全制度。

In addition, the lack or excess of sound, video and other equipment in the training ground will affect the hearing and vision, which will make the brain make wrong judgments. Insufficient or excessive light will make the nerve slow or too fast, which may cause sports injury. Therefore, in order to avoid the occurrence of injury, we should carefully check whether the equipment is safe before training, strengthen ideological safety education, and abide by various safety systems.

8. 气候条件不良

Bad Weather Conditions

气候条件的好坏也会导致某种运动性疾病或损伤的发生。如气温过高，容易产生疲劳和中暑；气温过低，易发生冻伤或出现肌肉僵硬，身体协调性下降而引起肌肉拉伤；潮湿高热的气候使人容易大量出汗，影响体内水盐代谢，可发生肌肉痉挛或虚脱。

Climate conditions can also lead to some sports diseases or injuries. If the temperature is too high, it is easy to lead to fatigue and heatstroke; if the temperature is too low, it is easy to lead to frostbite or muscle stiffness, and the decline of body coordination causes muscle strain; the humid and hot climate makes people sweat a lot, which affects the water and salt metabolism in the body, and can cause muscle spasm or collapse.

二、开放性软组织损伤和急性闭合性软组织损伤的处理

Section Two-Treatments of Open Soft Tissue Injury and Acute Closed Soft Tissue Injury

（一）开放性软组织损伤及处理

Open Soft Tissue Injury and Its Treatment

1. 擦伤

Abrasion

（1）概念

Definition

擦伤指机体表面与粗糙的物体相互摩擦而引起的皮肤表层损伤。

Abrasion is the superficial skin damage caused by the frictions between the body surface and rough objects.

（2）征象

Symptoms

伤口浅，面积大，边缘不整。

Shallow wounds with large areas and irregular margins.

表皮脱落，点状出血，组织液渗出。

The superficial skin falls off with punctate hemorrhage and interstitial fluid exudations.

无感染时，伤口易干燥结痂而愈合。伤口感染后易化脓，有较稠的渗出液。

Easy to heal by becoming dry and scabby without infections, but with thicker exudates if being infected.

（3）处理原则

Principles of Treatment

创口浅、面积小的擦伤：用生理盐水清洗后直接外涂2%的碘酊，无须包扎让其暴露在空气中即可。

Shallow, minor abrasions: clean out the wound with NS and apply 2% iodine tincture directly. It's okay to expose it in air without bandage.

创口内有异物及创口较深、污染严重的擦伤：及时就医。

Abrasions with foreign bodies in the wound: wash the wound with NS or tape water. Disinfect the wound with hydrogen peroxide and with 75% alcohol around the wound. After that apply sulfanilamide powder or aseptic dressing to it.

关节部位的擦伤：经消毒后，上消炎软膏或抗生素软膏，并用无菌敷料覆盖，一般不用暴露疗法。

Articular abrasions: apply an antiphlogistic cream or antibiotic cream and cover it with aseptic dressing after disinfection. Generally we don't use exposure therapy.

2. 裂伤、刺伤、切伤

Laceration, Sting and Cut

（1）概念

Definition

裂伤指身体受钝性暴力打击引起的皮肤、皮下组织撕裂。运动中头部裂伤最多，约占整个裂伤的61%，其中额部和面部居多。如篮球运动中，眉弓被对方肘部碰撞即可引起眉际裂伤。

Laceration is the tear of skin and subcutaneous tissue caused by blunt, violent blows. Cephalosome laceration is the most common laceration in sports, holding a proportion of about 61% of the total laceration, most on the foreheads and the faces. In a basketball game, a hit on the eye brow by an elbow can cause supercilia laceration.

刺伤指尖锐细物刺穿皮肤及皮下组织器官的损伤。

Sting is the injury caused by sharp, slender objects piercing the skin and subcutaneous tissue.

切伤指锐器切入皮肤及皮下组织所致的损伤。

Cut is the injury caused by sharp instruments cutting into skin and subcutaneous tissue.

（2）征象

Symptoms

裂伤：裂伤的伤口边缘不整，组织损伤广泛，出血多。

Laceration: the margin of the lacerating wound is irregular, with more bleeding and wider tissue injury.

刺伤：刺伤的伤口细小，但较深，可能伤及深部组织或器官，或者将异物带入伤口深处，容易引起感染。例如田径运动中鞋钉与标枪的刺伤。

Sting: slender but deep wound, which may hurt deep tissues and organs or take foreign objects deep into the wound, which is easy to cause infection. In track and field athletics, the injuries caused by hobnails and javelins are examples of stings.

切伤：切伤的伤口边缘整齐，伤口深，出血多。

Cut: the margin of the cut injury is regular, with more bleeding and deeper wound.

（3）处理原则

Principles of Treatment

注意检查伤口，观察污染情况；对于创口浅、面积小的损伤，可用生理盐水洗净伤口，75%的酒精或碘伏消毒，局部涂擦红紫药水，不用覆盖；如果伤口创面深且大时，应尽快前往医院清创、止血、缝合创口，做进一步治疗。

We need to check the wounds and observe the condition of pollution. For tiny, shallow wounds, we can clean them up with NS and disinfect with 75% alcohol or iodophor. Apply methylis violaceum or mercurochrome topically without coverage. If the wound is deep and large, we should go to a hospital as soon as possible.

（二）闭合性软组织损伤及处理

Closed soft Tissue Injury and Its Treatment

1. 概念

Definition

闭合性软组织损伤是指局部皮肤完整不开放，并且损伤时的出血积聚在组织内的损伤，有急性和慢性损伤两种。生活中常见的有崴伤、挫伤、肌肉拉伤、关节韧带拉伤等。

Closed soft tissue injury is the trauma with blood accumulating inside the tissues without tears on the skin. It is divided into acute and chronic wounds. The common symptoms include sprains, bruises, muscle strains and articular ligament strains, etc.

2. 成因

Cause of Formation

一般受伤的原因是运动中受钝力作用，肌肉猛烈收缩，导致关节活动超越正常范围或劳损，因此在对抗性较强的体育运动中更容易发生。

The most common causes of closed soft tissue injury is the fierce muscle contractions caused by blunt forces in sports. It can cause muscle actions beyond normal range or muscle strains so that it happens more easily in competitive sports.

3. 闭合性损伤的处理

Treatment of Closed Injury

（1）病理变化

Pathological Change

组织血肿和水肿，局部红、肿、热、痛和功能障碍。

Hematomas and edemas in tissues with localized swellings, heat, pains and dysfunction.

（2）处理原则

Principle

制动、止血、镇痛、防肿及减轻炎症。

Immobilization, hemostasis, postoperative analgesia, anti-edema and inflammation reduction.

（3）处理建议

Treatment Suggestions

在受伤后应当立刻冷敷、加压包扎并抬高伤肢。如果条件允许，可以使用外敷创伤药，达到消肿、止痛和减轻炎症的效果。如果疼痛过于剧烈应及时就医。

After getting hurt, you need to apply ice and pressure bandaging to it and lift up the injured limb. If conditions allow, vulnerary for external application can be applied to do swell, relieve pain and reduce inflammation. If there's sharp pain, you should go to a hospital.

（三）运动损伤一般应急处置原则

Basic Principles of Treatments for Athletic Injuries

RICE原则是运动损伤后要尽快遵守的康复原则的英文首字缩写的组合，它可以把疼痛、肿胀和发炎的程度降到最低，缩短恢复的时间。

RICE principle is a combination of acronyms which refers to the principals of treatments which need to be observed as soon as possible after athletic injuries. It can minimize the degree of pain, edema and inflammation, and shorten the recovery period.

1. 休息

Rest

指应停止一切活动以避免受伤部位进一步损伤和出血。休息时，可以在不发生损伤的前提下，先将受伤部位归位到起始状态。在此期间，受伤部位不可以承重，通常要求伤者坐着或躺着。受伤部位在48小时以内不允许抵抗外力，以限制瘢痕组织的增生。

It means that all activities should be ceased to prevent injured parts from further damage and bleeding. When at rest we can put the injured parts back to right positon on the premise of no further damage. During this period, the injured parts cannot bear load. Usually, the injured should be asked to sit or lie. Within 48 hours the injured part cannot resist external forces to limit the hyperplasia of scar tissues.

2. 冰敷

Ice Compress

冰敷，是指用布包好冰块敷在受伤部位，来减缓和冷却流向受伤部位的血液，以减轻炎症。需要注意的是冰块不能与皮肤直接接触。实践表明，冰敷还有缓解疼痛的作用，可以减轻伤痛带来的肌肉痉挛和肌肉紧张。

Ice compress refers to the use of cloth wrapping ice applied to the injured part, so as to slow down and cool the blood flow to the injured part, in order to reduce inflammation. It should be noted that the ice should not be in direct contact with the skin. Practice shows that ice compress can also relieve pain, and can reduce muscle spasm and muscle tension caused by injury.

3. 加压包扎

Compression

在受伤后，应尽快对受伤部位进行加压包扎，压迫血管止血，尽量减少患部出血。包扎时将一块硬物垫在绷带下，压住伤口。不可以对受伤部位的四周都进行压迫，会阻塞血液流通。加压包扎可以保持几天时间。

After getting injured, we should compress the wounded part as soon as possible to reduce bleeding. When wrapping up, we should mat a hard object under the bandage to compress the wound. Never compress the whole surroundings of the wound, otherwise the blood circulation may be blocked. Compression can last for several days.

4. 抬高

Elevation

抬高受伤部位会帮助静脉和淋巴回流，减少血液循环至伤处，避免肿胀，促进恢复。任何受伤的部位都应该支撑起来抬高，时间越长越好，直到肿胀消除。

Elevating the wounded part will help the reflux of vena and lymph. Reduce the blood circulation to the wound to avoid swelling and promote recovery. Any injured part should be elevated as long as possible until the swellings diminish.

三、运动损伤的防治措施

Section Three–Prevention and Treatment of Sports Injuries

在体育运动过程中，运动损伤的出现不仅存在偶然原因，同时也存在一些必然原因，如运动、管理、监督、组织等方面的不合理，都有可能导致关节损伤发生率的激增。

In sports, there are not only accidental reasons, but also some inevitable reasons, such as unreasonable sports, management, supervision, organization and so on, which may lead to a sharp increase in the incidence of joint injury.

（一）强化安全知识教育

Strengthen Safety Knowledge Education

1. 加强安全知识宣传

Strengthen the Publicity of Safety Knowledge

通过多途径、多样化学习，加强运动安全知识教育。如理论学习、海报宣传等，使学生掌握运动过程中可能产生的运动伤病的知识及提高预防意识。准确掌握医疗保健相关知识，根据学生的运动情况、运动意识等做好相应的宣传正确运动工作；定期开展医疗卫生理论知识、运动技巧的讲座。

Through diversified learning, teachers should promote the education of sports safety knowledge by theoretical study, poster publicity, etc. In this way, students can master the knowledge of sports injuries and improve the awareness of prevention. Meanwhile, teachers should grasp the relevant knowledge of medical and health care accurately, do the corresponding propaganda according to the students' sports situation and sports consciousness, and carry out the correct sports mode. Last but not least, teachers should organize some lectures on medical and health theory knowledge and sports skills regularly.

2. 做好运动前安全警示（提醒）

Safety Warning Before Exercise (Notice)

在做高强度的运动之前，体能训练的各个部门需要相互协作，做好对学生的健康运动以及体育训练运动损伤预防知识的讲解宣传工作,从而有效提升学生对于体育训练运动损伤预防措施的理解与掌握能力,促使学生在训练过程中做到自我保护。

Before doing high-intensity sports, the various departments of physical training need to cooperate with each other to do a good job in explaining and publicizing knowledge of students' health and sports injury prevention in sports training, so as to effectively improve students' understanding and mastering ability of sports injury prevention measures in sports training, and promote students to achieve self-protection in the process of training.

（二）科学合理地组织训练

Organize Training Scientifically and Reasonably

1. 做好运动前的准备活动

Get Ready for Sports

运动之前的准备活动的目的在于提升中枢系统的兴奋状态,促使其保持最佳的水平;强化不同器官的运动功能,从而克服功能相关性惰性表现,提升组织的温度并改善血液循环,提升肌肉力量与弹性,强化肌肉组织与神经系统的条件反射效果,为后续的训练奠定基础。准备活动量需要按照个体的机能进行适当调节,在兴奋性比较低或者是气温比较低的情况下,准备活动的时间应当适当延长,以身体发热与稍微出汗为标准。准备活动的内容应当按照教学、训练或者是竞赛的具体内容进行选择,不仅需要有一般性的准备活动,还需安排针对性的专项准备性活动。准备活动结束和正式训练或竞赛之间的间隔时间应当以5分钟以内为最佳。

The purpose of preparatory activities before exercise is to improve the excited state of the central system and keep it at the best level. Strengthen the motor function of different organs, so as to overcome the performance of function related inertia, improve the tissue temperature and blood circulation, enhance muscle strength and elasticity, strengthen the conditioned reflex effect of muscle tissue and nervous system, and lay a foundation for subsequent training. The amount of preparatory activity needs to be adjusted according to the individual's function. In the case of low excitability or low temperature, the time of preparatory activity should be extended appropriately, with slight sweating as the standard. The preparatory activities should be selected according to the specific content of teaching, training or competition. It needs not only general preparatory activities, but also specific preparatory activities. The interval between the end of preparatory activities and formal training or competition should be less than 5 minutes.

2. 科学合理地制订运动计划

Make Exercise Plan Scientifically and Reasonably

体能训练过程中，应当有意识、科学地组织训练，使训练本身不仅可以实现对学生体能的强化，同时也可以保障训练不超出学生的身体负荷能力，最大限度地预防体育训练运动损伤事件的发生。科学组织训练需要从多个角度着手。首先，在训练开始之前需要按照学生的实际身体素质制订具体的训练计划，同时按照不同训练的科目内容、时间、强度等进行针对性的规划，尽可能规避下肢的高强度集中性训练，用循序渐进的训练方式强化学生的身体机能。在每天的训练中还需要根据当天的训练要求对学生实行肌群准备训练，让学生以更好的身体状态参与到运动当中。

In physical training, teachers should organize the training consciously and scientifically, so that the training can not only strengthen the students' physical fitness, but also ensure that the training does not exceed the students' physical load capacity, and prevent the occurrence of sports injury events in sports training to the greatest extent. Scientific organized training needs to be conducted from many aspects. First of all, before the start of training, it is necessary to formulate specific training plans according to the actual physical quality of students, and make targeted planning according to the content, time and intensity of different training subjects, so as to avoid the high-intensity concentrated training of lower limbs as far as possible, and strengthen the physical functions of students in a step-by-step way. In the daily training, we also need to carry out muscle group preparation training for students according to the training requirements of the day, so that students can participate in sports in a better physical state.

（三）改进运动理念

Improve Thoughts of Sports

应用运动创伤和体疗康复保障体质健康。运动创伤简单而言属于骨科创伤的分支科目，其主要是指学生在体能训练锻炼期间，运动系统所形成的一种急性或慢性损伤，这一损伤的诊疗主要是围绕着学生的骨骼发育、多方面机体功能的创伤等内容为主。另外，还需要按照运动创伤所形成的规律、机理等进行针对分析，在运动期间可能存在各种运动损伤，普遍都和不同运动项目的不同特征有直接关联性。例如，学生在训练过程中最容易损伤的部位是踝关节，所以训练期间需要高度重视对踝关节的保护，提升运动技巧以及运动的安全性，降低损伤风险。体疗康复则是运动损伤之后的治疗干预措施，主要目的在于修复或重建损失的运动功能。具体而言就是医务人员合理应用各种先进的器械设备或相关技术，针对运动员因为损伤而失去的部分功能进行修复，按照不同损伤情况制订具体的治疗干预方式，同时做好相应的运动处方调整，降低再次损伤的风险。损伤初期以积极治疗为主；干预期间做好后续训练的调整与优化，规避损伤再次发生；训练期间合理地应用保护带等工具。

Applying sports trauma recovery and physical therapy rehabilitation to ensure physical health. Sports trauma is a branch of orthopedic trauma, which mainly refers to an acute or chronic injury formed by the sports system during students' physical training. The diagnosis and treatment of this injury mainly focuses on students' bone development and injuries of various body functions. In addition, we also need to analyze the rules and mechanism of sports injuries. There may be various sports injuries during exercise, which are generally directly related to the different characteristics of different sports. For example, the most vulnerable part of students in the process of training is the ankle joint, so we need to attach great importance to the protection of ankle joint during training, improve sports skills and safety, and reduce the risk of injury. Physical therapy rehabilitation is the treatment intervention after sports injury, mainly aimed at repairing or reconstructing the lost motor function. Specifically, the medical staff should make reasonable use of various advanced equipment or related technologies to repair some functions lost by athletes due to injury, formulate specific treatment interventions according to different injury conditions, and make corresponding adjustment of sports prescription to reduce the risk of another injury. In the early stage of injury, active treatment is the main method; during the intervention, follow-up training should be adjusted and optimized to avoid injury recurrence. Protective belt should be used reasonably during training.

（四）运动营养的合理调配

Reasonable Allocation of Sports Nutrition

在运动与体能练习时，不仅需要掌握相应的运动机能，同时还需要掌握部分运动营养相关知识，为自身提供营养支持，合理地制定并落实运动营养方案，促使自身的身体素质持续增强，帮助机体快速恢复，及时补充所需要的营养。但是，必须高度重视不同营养物质对于身体素质的影响，高度重视营养物的选择合理性、摄入量的适宜性，如果摄入不足会导致学生机体功能无法发挥，过多会导致身体负担提高。对此，运动营养必须合理、有针对性且科学，才能为身体健康提供可靠支持。针对频发的运动损伤情况需要做好全面性的分析，并从营养搭配的角度进行预防控制，从而降低运动损伤的负面影响。

In sports and physical training, we need to master not only the corresponding sports function, but also some sports nutrition related knowledge, provide nutrition support for ourselves, reasonably formulate and implement sports nutrition program, promote our own physical quality, help the body recover quickly and timely supplement the needed nutrition. However, we must attach great importance to the influence of different nutrients on physical fitness, the rationality of the choice of nutrients and the suitability of intake. If the intake is insufficient, the body function of students will not be able to perform, and excess of nutrition will lead to the increase of body burden. Therefore, nutrition intake for doing sports must be reasonable, targeted and scientific in order to provide reliable support for health. In view of the frequent sports injury, we need to do a comprehensive analysis, and prevent and control it from the perspective of nutrition collocation, so as to reduce the negative impact of sports injury.

（五）合理选购运动装备

Reasonable Selection of Sports Equipment

选择合适的装备也是加强保护的重要途径之一。如选择合适的服装和鞋子，选择相应的护具以保护容易受伤的部位。从踝关节的护踝到肘关节的护肘，从举重时用的腰带到不起眼的健美裤等，这些看似细小的运动护具，却能够在我们平时锻炼的过程中为肌肉和关节分担外来的压力和冲击。而各种关节是运动中最容易损伤的部位，关节过伸或过屈都有可能对肌腱造成损害，除做好热身运动外，适当佩戴护具能在很大程度上避免肌腱过度拉伸。护具可以让关节和肌肉在正常范围内运动，而超常运动是造成损伤的重要原因之一。对于参加体育锻炼的人来说，最好的护具就是绷带和胶布，两者与肌肉的结合程度最紧密，也能够最好地保护肌肉和关节。打篮球的时候戴上护腕、护膝、护踝，踢足球的时候加上护腿板，护肘、护腕是打网球、羽毛球、乒乓球必不可少的用品，这些微不足道的小护具，在关键时刻却能为保护我们的身体帮上大忙。

Choosing the right equipment is also one of important ways to strengthen protection. For example, choose appropriate clothing, shoes and appropriate protective gear to protect the vulnerable parts such as ankle joint and elbow joint protection. From belt used in weightlifting to humble bodybuilding pants, etc, these sports protectors are seemingly small but can share the external pressure and impact for muscles and joints during our normal exercise. All kinds of joints are the most vulnerable parts, and joint hyperextension or hyperflexion may cause damage to the tendon. In addition to good warm-up exercise, appropriately wearing protective equipment can largely avoid tendon overstretching. Protectors can make joints and muscles move in normal range, and abnormal movement is one of the important reasons for injury. For people who take part in physical exercise, the best protective gear is bandage and adhesive tape. The combination of bandage and adhesive tape is the closest, and they can also best protect muscles and joints. When playing basketball, wear wrist, knee and ankle protectors, and when playing football, add leg protectors. Elbow and wrist protectors are essential supplies for playing tennis, badminton and table tennis. These little protectors may help us to protect our body at the critical moment.

（六）完善自我医务监督工作

Improve Self-Medical Supervision

医务监督是指用医学的方法对运动参与者的机能及健康进行监督和协助，使其运动符合身心发展规律，科学合理地进行，进而预防运动中的一些危险因素对参与者造成伤害。通过自我医学监督，可以有效地利用体育手段促进自身身心健康的发展，避免运动伤病的发生，人们在运动中一旦出现不适现象，可及时调整锻炼与训练计划，进行相应的治疗和康复。这是掌握必要的自我医务监督知识和方法，提高自我保护能力的重要体现。

Medical supervision refers to the use of medical methods to supervise and assist the function and health of sports participants, so as to make their training process conform to the law of physical and mental development, scientific and reasonable, and then prevent some risk factors in sports from causing harm to the participants. Through self-medical supervision, we can effectively use sports to promote the development of our physical and mental health and avoid the occurrence of sports injuries. When you feel discomfort in sports, you can timely adjust the exercise and training plan, and carry out the corresponding treatment and rehabilitation. This is an important embodiment of mastering the necessary knowledge and methods of self-medical supervision and improving the ability of self-protection.

思考

Questions

1. 请结合本章内容，为中老年人预防高血压提供生活方式上的建议。

Please provide advice on lifestyle for middle-aged and elderly people to prevent hypertension in conjunction with the content of this chapter.

2. 请根据糖尿病的运动管理内容，为糖尿病患者设计一份运动处方。

Please design an exercise prescription for diabetic patients based on the content of sports management.

3. 血脂异常可以通过哪些方式加以改善？你认为什么样的生活方式有助于保持良好的血脂水平？

In what ways can dyslipidemia be improved? What kind of lifestyle do you think that that helps maintain good blood lipid levels?

4. 骨质疏松症的健康管理分为哪几方面？你认为哪一方面最容易被忽视？并尝试就此给出建议。

What are aspects of the health management of osteoporosis? Which aspect do you think is most easily overlooked? And try to give suggestions on this.

5. 本章介绍的慢性疾病所带来的危害有哪些共性？如何针对这些共性进行健康管理？

What are commonalities in the harm caused by the chronic diseases introduced in this chapter? How to conduct health management in the light of these commonalities?

6. 如果你在运动中不慎扭伤了脚踝，应该如何正确处理？请简单说说有哪些步骤。

If you sprain your ankle while training, how to deal with it correctly? What are the steps?

7. 造成运动损伤的原因包括哪些？请结合亲身经历谈谈自己的理解。

What are causes of sports injuries? Please talk about your understanding with your own experience.

参考文献
REFERENCE

［1］Peter R. Kongstvedt. Essentials of Managed Health Care-Jones & Bartlett Learning. Jones & Bartlett Publishers, 2007.

［2］宋卉, 刘华. 健康管理概览［M］. 北京：中国轻工业出版社, 2016.

［3］张庆军, 祝淑珍, 李俊琳. 实用健康管理学［M］. 北京：科学出版社, 2017.

［4］王培玉. 健康管理学［M］. 北京：北京大学医学出版社, 2012.

［5］郭清. 健康管理学概论［M］. 北京：人民卫生出版社, 2011.

［6］廖岚岚. 构建社区健康素养教育学的辩证思考［J］. 工程技术研究, 2019, 1（17）:197-201.

［7］单紫徽, 喻龙, 宋绍鹏. 构建高校学生体质健康管理模式的措施［J］. 当代体育科技, 2020, 10（5）:129-130.

［8］杨春玲, 冯晶军, 袁玮等. 一对一健康管理对改善亚健康人群患慢性病风险性的影响［J］. 中华现代护理杂志, 2010, 16（12）:1369-1372.

［9］周迎松, 陈小平. 六大营养素与体能［J］. 中国体育科技, 2014（04）:93-103.

［10］权永妮. 七大营养素与人体健康［J］. 科技信息，2012（36）:168+170.

［11］黄强, 舒婷, 王钏等. 浅谈膳食纤维与健康［J］. 食品安全导刊, 2018（27）:75.

［12］张前锋. 体能类运动员的强力营养素补充［J］. 科技视界, 2019

（19）:133-133.

[13] 宋永范,彭雪涵,林黛茜.不同项目运动员营养补充特点研究综述[J].福建体育科技,2012,31（6）:35-37.

[14] 蒋碧艳,祝蓓里.上海市大中学生的心理健康及其与体育锻炼的关系[J].心理科学,1997（03）:235-238+287.

[15] 牛亚光.体育活动对大学生心理健康的干预[J].体育科技文献通报,2019,27（11）:168-170.

[16] 季浏.体育锻炼与心理健康[M].上海：华东师范大学出版社,2006.

[17] 吴晓薇,黄玲,何晓琴等.大学生社交焦虑与攻击、抑郁：情绪调节自我效能感的中介作用[J].中国临床心理学杂志,2015,23（05）:50-53.

[18] 徐霞.社会性体格焦虑的测量及其与身体锻炼之间关系的研究[D].上海：华东师范大学,2003.

[19] 李佳川.体育锻炼对降低大学生自卑感的影响及其心理机制研究[D].上海：华东师范大学,2009.

[20] 夏维波,章振林,林华等.原发性骨质疏松症诊疗指南（2017）[J].中国骨质疏松杂志,2019,25（03）:281-309.

[21] Z.J. Xu, W. Qi, Y. Liu . Effect of warm needling plus oral medication on blood lipids in cerebral infarction patients [J]. Journal of Acupuncture and Tuina Science, 2017, 15（2）:115-119.

[22] M.Y. Ma, J.F. Jiang, X.Y. Zhou, etal. Influence of suspended moxibustion on the biochemical markers of patients with hyperlipidemia [J]. Journal of Acupuncture and Tuina Science, 2012, 10（6）:364-367.

[23] 苗桂珍,崔赵丽.与"糖"同行——中西医结合防治糖尿病[M].北京：人民卫生出版社,2017.

[24] 刘铮然,王素华.全科医学导论[M].北京：科学出版社,2016.

[25] 曹霞,谢秀梅,杨娉婷等.基于PDCA模式对功能社区正常高值血压

人群实施健康教育的效果［J］.中华护理杂志,2014,49（04）:485-491.

［26］杨光福.血脂异常患者六大注意事项［J］.医师在线,2016,6（5）:32-33.

［27］陈茜,薛勇,宋晓峰等.糖尿病及糖尿病心血管并发症患者肠道菌群的特征［J］.微生物学报,2019,59（9）:1660-1673.

［28］陶涛,袁静.血压、血脂、血糖及肾功能不同水平对老年高血压心血管事件的影响［J］.河北医药,2017,2（39）:45-48.

［29］孙莉敏,胡永善,吴毅.运动锻炼对Ⅱ型糖尿病患者血脂与体质指标的影响［J］.中国运动医学杂志,2002（01）:51-53+94.

［30］马远征,王以朋,刘强等.中国老年骨质疏松症诊疗指南（2018）［J］.中国实用内科杂志,2019,39（01）:38-61.

［31］李洋,陈明慧,洪克敏等.中低强度体育锻炼对社区高血压患者康复疗效分析［J］.中国运动医学杂志,2002（05）:479-483.

［32］中华医学会内分泌学分会.高尿酸血症和痛风治疗的中国专家共识［J］.中华内分泌代谢杂志,2013,29（11）:913-920.

［33］李斌,郭均涛,王宏等.体质量指数、腰臀比、体脂百分率评价青少年肥胖的研究［J］.重庆医学,2014（34）:83-85+88.

［34］黄国梅,熊丰,曾燕等.腰围、腰围/身高比值和腰臀比与儿童青少年血压的相关性研究［J］.重庆医科大学学报,2009（03）:110-114.

［35］朱琳,陈佩杰.能量消耗测量方法及其应用［J］.中国运动医学杂志,2011（06）:72-77.

［36］李冲,史曙生.健康青年男性两种力量负荷抗阻训练能量消耗的推算［J］.中国运动医学杂志,2019（5）:364-371.

［37］郭永峰.用心率测量监控运动训练强度方法的探讨［J］.青海师范大学学报（自然科学版）,2006（3）:102-103.

［38］温搏.中国传统体育养生中英双语教程［M］.北京:北京师范大学出版社,2015.

［39］白震民. 中医康复疗法双语指南［M］. 北京：北京体育大学出版社, 2013.

［40］刘洪福, 安海燕, 王长虹等. 健身气功—八段锦健心功效实验探讨［J］. 武汉体育学院学报, 2008（01）：54-57+77.

［41］周小青. 健身气功—八段锦对中老年人身体形态、生理机能及血脂的影响［D］. 北京：北京体育大学, 2003.

［42］陈辉, 周亚娜. 八段锦对原发性高血压患者血压和血清超敏C反应蛋白的影响［J］. 中国康复医学杂志, 2012, 27（02）：178-179.

［43］M.P. Garofalo. Eight Section Brocade Chi Kung［EB/OL］. http://www.egreenway.com/taichichuan/esb.htm, 2006.

［44］陈亚军, 吕雅杰. 综合评估儿童行为模式 提升学生健康水平［J］. 中国学校卫生, 2019, 40（12）：1761-1766.

［45］祝园园. 2018年任城区健康教育和健康促进现况研究［D］. 山东：山东大学, 2019.

［46］周珊宇, 温贤忠, 陈嘉斌等. 广东省重点职业病监测情况与职业健康风险评估［J］. 中国公共卫生, 2019, 35（05）：549-553.

［47］丁兰君, 赵丽中, 王媛等. 中国结直肠癌健康风险评估模型研究［J］. 中国慢性病预防与控制, 2018, 26（05）：325-328.

［48］倪睿. 杭州市中小学生体质健康调查及健康危险因素研究［D］. 上海：复旦大学, 2012.

［49］刘洋. 健康管理视角下商业健康保险风险控制研究［D］. 黑龙江中医药大学, 2019.

［50］Griffith Kevin N, Jones David K, Bor Jacob H, Sommers Benjamin D. Changes in Health Insurance Coverage, Access to Care, and Income-Based Disparities Among US Adults［J］. Health affairs（Project Hope）, 2020, 39（2）:27-32.

［51］朱铭来, 奎潮. 论商业健康保险在新医疗保障体系中的地位［J］.

保险研究, 2009（1）: 70-76.

［52］顾昕. 中国商业健康保险的现状与发展战略［J］. 保险研究, 2009（11）: 26-33.

［53］许志伟. 我国健康管理与健康保险结合的意义［J］. 中华医学信息导报, 2006（12）: 6.

［54］王素改, 钟亚平. 高山滑雪运动损伤特征、影响因素及预防策略研究进展［J］. 武汉体育学院学报, 2019, 53（12）: 59-67.

［55］闫鹏宇, 张新安. 核心训练及其预防运动损伤的作用研究进展［J］. 沈阳体育学院学报, 2018, 37（03）: 83-88.

［56］周昕虔, 杨绛梅, 刘小学等. 女大学生户外健身登山运动损伤发生的特征研究［J］. 首都体育学院学报, 2015, 27（03）: 282-285.

［57］栾丽霞, 徐祥峰. 大学生网球运动损伤的调查研究［J］. 武汉体育学院学报, 2005（06）: 92-95.

［58］石大玲, 章爱珍. 我国大学生运动损伤调查及病因分析［J］. 武汉体育学院学报, 2004（03）: 52-53+55.